IMMUNOLOGIC METHODS
IN STEROID DETERMINATION

IMMUNOLOGIC METHODS
IN STEROID DETERMINATION

Fernand G. Péron
Burton V. Caldwell

Worcester Foundation for Experimental Biology
Shrewsbury, Massachusetts 01545

PLENUM PRESS • NEW YORK AND LONDON

Library of Congress Cataloging in Publication Data

Main entry under title:

Immunologic methods in steroid determination.

Based on a symposium held at the Worcester Foundation for Experimental Biology, Nov. 18-20, 1969.
Includes bibliographies.
1. Steroid hormones—Congresses. 2. Immunoglobulins—Congresses. 3. Immuno-specificity—Congresses. 4. Radioimmunoassay—Congresses. I. Péron, Fernand G., 1925-   ed. II. Caldwell, Burton V., ed. [DNLM: 1. Antigen-antibody reactions—Congresses. 2. Radioimmunoassay—Congresses. 3. Sex hormones—Analysis —Congresses. 4. Steroids—Analysis—Congresses. WK150 I33 1969]
QP572.S7I45   1974   612'.405   74-17058
ISBN-13: 978-1-4684-6053-7   e-ISBN-13: 978-1-4684-6051-3
DOI: 10.1007/ 978-1-4684-6051-3

© 1970 Plenum Press, New York
Softcover reprint of the hardcover 1st edition 1970
A Division of Plenum Publishing Corporation
227 West 17th Street, New York, N.Y. 10011

United Kingdom edition published by Plenum Press, London
A Division of Plenum Publishing Company, Ltd.
4a Lower John Street, London W1R 3PD, England

CONTRIBUTORS

GUY E. ABRAHAM   Worcester Foundation For Experimental Biology, Shrewsbury, Massachusetts 01545; Present address: Division of Endocrinology, Harbor General Hospital, Torrance, California 90509

SUMNER H. BURSTEIN   Worcester Foundation for Experimental Biology, Shrewsbury, Massachusetts 01545

BURTON V. CALDWELL   Worcester Foundation for Experimental Biology, Shrewsbury, Massachusetts 01545; Present address: Department of Obstetrics and Gynecology, Yale University Medical School, New Haven, Connecticut 06510

HSIU-WU CHUNG   Department of Obstetrics and Gynecology, The University of Texas, Southwestern Medical School at Dallas, Dallas, Texas 75234

MICHEL FERIN   The International Institute for the Study of Human Reproduction, Department of Obstetrics and Gynecology, Columbia University College of Physicians and Surgeons, New York, New York 10032

LAWRENCE GOODFRIEND   The Harry Webster Thorp Laboratories, Division of Immunochemistry and Allergy, McGill University Clinic, Royal Victoria Hospital, Montreal, Quebec, Canada

STANLEY J. GROSS   Department of Pathology, University of California, Irvine, California College of Medicine, Irvine, California 92664

ALLAN L. GROSSBERG   Roswell Park Memorial Institute, Buffalo, New York 14203

A. REES MIDGLEY, JR.   The Reproduction and Endocrinology Program of the Department of Pathology, University of Michigan, Ann Arbor, Michigan 48104

GEORGE MIKHAIL   Department of Obstetrics and Gynecology, The University of Texas, Southwestern Medical School at Dallas, Dallas, Texas 75234

GORDON D. NISWENDER   The Reproduction and Endocrinology Program of the Department of Pathology, The University of Michigan, Ann Arbor, Michigan 48104

WILLIAM ODELL   Division of Endocrinology, Harbor General Hospital, Torrance, California 90509

DAVID PRESSMAN   Roswell Park Memorial Institute, Buffalo, New York 14203

JOSEPH RAZIANO   Department of Obstetrics and Gynecology, Columbia University College of Physicians and Surgeons, New York, New York 10032

REX J. SCARAMUZZI   Worcester Foundation for Experimental Biology, Shrewsbury, Massachusetts 01545

ALEC SEHON   Department of Immunology, The University of Manitoba, Winnipeg, Manitoba, Canada

ANTONIO TEMPONE   Department of Obstetrics and Gynecology, Columbia University College of Physicians and Surgeons, New York, New York 10032; Present address: University of Buenos Aires School of Medicine, Buenos Aires, Argentina

IAN H. THORNEYCROFT   Worcester Foundation for Experimental Biology, Shrewsbury, Massachusetts 01545; Present address: Department of Obstetrics and Gynecology, Livingston Research Center, University of Southern California, School of Medicine, Los Angeles, California 90033

STEPHEN A. TILLSON   Worcester Foundation for Experimental Biology, Shrewsbury, Massachusetts 01545

RAYMOND L. VANDE WIELE   Department of Obstetrics and Gynecology, Columbia University College of Physicians and Surgeons, New York, New York 10032

ACKNOWLEDGMENTS

This volume is based on a symposium held at the Worcester Foundation for Experimental Biology, November 18-20, 1969. We would like to acknowledge the following companies who supported this symposium financially and in no small measure contributed to its success: Abbott Laboratories; Alza Corporation; Armour Pharmaceutical Company; Astra Pharmaceutical Products, Inc.; Ayerst Laboratories; Charles River Breeding Laboratories; CIBA Pharmaceutical Company; Hoffmann-La Roche Foundation; Eli Lilly and Company; Mason Research Institute; Merck & Company, Inc.; Miles Laboratories, Inc.; New England Nuclear Corp.; Organon Inc.; Ortho Research Foundation; Charles Pfizer & Company, Inc.; Schering Corporation; G. D. Searle & Co.; Smith, Kline & French Laboratories; E. R. Squibb & Sons; Sterling-Winthrop Research Institute; Syntex Corporation.

We would also like to thank all Worcester Foundation personnel who gave of their valuable time before and during the symposium. A special vote of thanks is given to Mrs. Carol McMullin for secretarial help and to Mrs. Margaret Flack for editorial assistance.

PREFACE

The two main goals of the symposium upon which this volume is based were 1) to cement together knowledge presently available in the field of antibodies to steroids and obtainable only under separate covers in different journals and books, and 2) to present new data which could lead to a more complete understanding of physiologic phenomena like those occurring during the menstrual cycle, or to the elucidation of the mechanisms involved in steroid-protection interaction, or to the practical application of immunologic techniques to measurements of steroid hormones. These techniques are extremely sensitive and can measure levels of steroid on the same order of magnitude as the radioisotope methods. However, the latter are much more laborious and costly which limits their use in many cases to the research laboratory. But the immunologic techniques generally classified as radioimmunoassay, are fraught with difficulties and problems which must be overcome.

Fortunately, perhaps, the subject of immunologic techniques as applied to steroid determination is the child of radioimmunoassay of proteins, so to speak. Many of the problems which confront the former have been resolved in the latter instance. Thus, we are in an advantageous position because we are aware of the biologic and technical problems of the earlier radioimmunoassay techniques. Similar experiences have been reported in the book about the use of immunologic techniques for determination of steroid hormones.

Therefore the task of the participants, in their presentations and discussions, and of those entering the discussions was one of presenting findings permitting everyone attending to share their experiences which could eventually lead to solutions of the difficulties and problems involved in immunologic techniques. It need be mentioned in passing that the final methods used must satisfy the requirements of specificity, reproducibility, precision, and sensitivity. Other points which should be considered are rapidity, simplicity, and cost. I believe that the immunologic techniques already have the latter attributes and that many determinations can be carried out in hundreds of samples much more simply, rapidly and at much less cost than with the accurate, precise, and sensitive radioisotope assays.

Thus, a rapid gain in popularity of the immunologic techniques for steroid determinations is foreseen. Even the most "old-fashioned" scientist, as encrusted as he may be in older concepts of methodology, cannot help but notice from occasional furtive listening that styles are changing in methodology. If the contributors have been able to present their work here in such a manner as to support the above prophecy as well as stress the requirements for the application of good immunologic techniques, I venture to say that the proceedings of this symposium will be of great help in guiding students and researchers alike in modern immunologic techniques as applied to steroid hormone determinations.

Quite apart from the uses of antibodies to steroids in quantitation procedures are the studies employing immunization of animals against steroids as a means of elucidating the complex interrelationship between steroid hormones and pituitary and gonadal function. The potential of this new approach was evident to all as the results of investigations involving the neutralization of steroids in vivo were presented. Although this technique is in its infancy its application to some long-standing problems has provided answers unavailable by older methods.

Finally, we will have amply justified the preparation of this volume if, out of the presentations and discussions, everyone obtains an immediate full measure of information. This information will mean new approaches to old and more recent problems and hopefully lead to their solutions. I would like to feel that the approaches we have taken not only do justice to the subject at hand, but honor two men, Drs. Hudson Hoagland and Gregory Pincus, who were co-founders of the Worcester Foundation for Experimental Biology. Dr. Pincus' untimely death in 1967 saddened many people all over the world and had its impact on the scientific community at large and especially on our own. If my efforts are in any way partly responsible in having made this book successful, I would like to dedicate them to the memory of Dr. Gregory Pincus.

Fernand Péron

CONTENTS

Part III   The Use of Antibodies to Steroids in Physiologic Studies

IMMUNOLOGIC METHODS
IN STEROID DETERMINATION

PART I
Chemical and Immunologic Aspects of Antibodies to Steroids

1

STRUCTURAL BASIS OF
ANTIBODY SPECIFICITY

David Pressman and Allan L. Grossberg

Roswell Park Memorial Institute*
Buffalo, New York

INTRODUCTION

Immunologic methods for steroid determination depend on the ability of antibodies directed against a steroid determinant group to react preferentially with that particular steroid. The specificity of the reaction depends on a complementary fit of the combining site of the antibody with the steroid of interest.

Several views of the estradiol-17β-succinyl group are shown in Figure 1. It would be expected that many different types of antibody molecules would react with this group, each type of antibody being complementary to a different part of the group. Such a heterogeneous population of antibodies reacting with a particular hapten has been shown for several systems, such as the anti-*p*-azobenzoate systems and the anti-azoisophthaloyl-glycine-D,L-leucine systems (Pressman and Grossberg, 1968, p. 150.) These antibodies can be fractionated with respect to their specificities. Furthermore, in analogy with antibodies against other haptens, it would be expected that the anti-estradiol-17β-succinyl antibodies formed by

This work was supported in part by Grant No. AI-3962 from the National Institute of Allergy and Infectious Diseases.
* A unit of the New York State Department of Health.

1

individual animals would differ greatly from animal to animal in specificity and in combining constant. It would also be expected that the antibodies produced by an individual animal would be made up primarily of just a few different, distinct antibody populations, as discussed later.

The fact that·the antibodies produced by individual animals show differences in specificity becomes particularly important in the selection of antibodies for assay purposes. These should be selected by assaying the

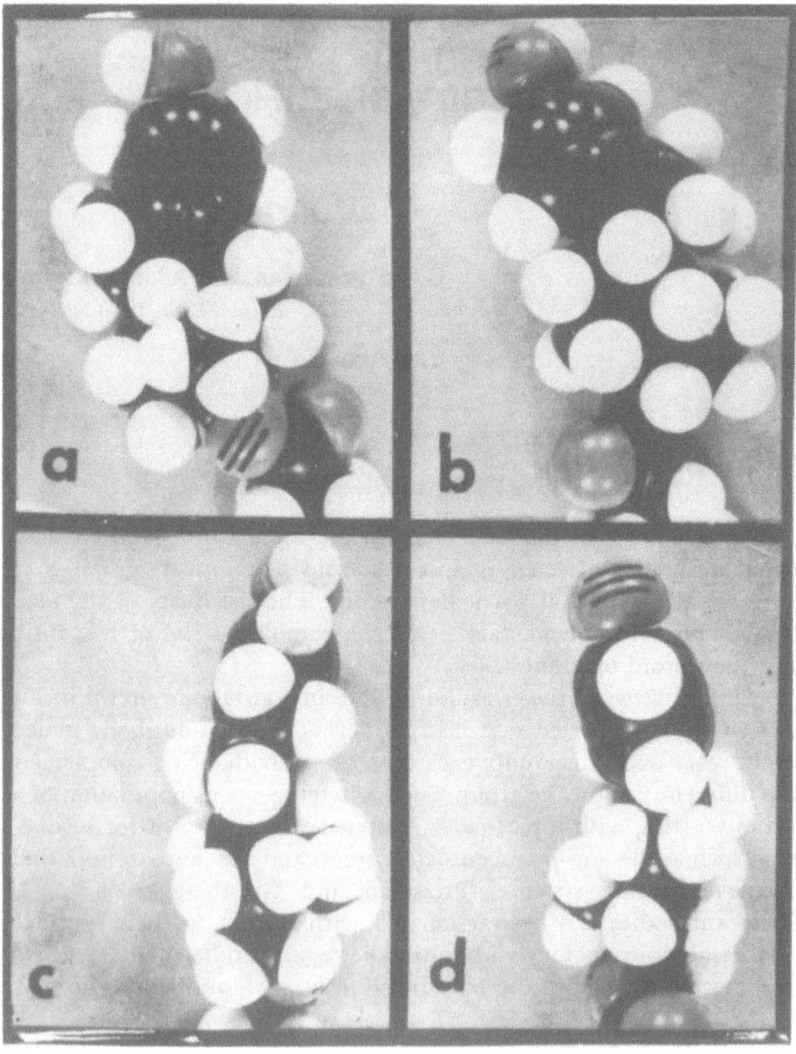

Fig. 1.   Various steric aspects of the estradiol-17β-succinyl group.

antibodies from one animal rather than pooling sera from several animals, since a particular antiserum may have important selective properties, and the antibodies responsible for these properties would only be diluted by a mixture of sera from other animals.

The specificity of the combining site of any particular antibody molecule is determined by its configuration and composition and, thus, ultimately by the primary sequences of the component polypeptide chains. Again, by analogy with antibodies against other haptens, it would be expected that the antibody molecules which react selectively with one particular steroid would not all have the same amino acid sequence. Indeed, it would be expected that many different antibody molecules, each with a different structure, would be capable of combining with a particular steroid group.

Antibodies, even of a single globulin type, which are capable of combining with a particular hapten have been shown to differ with regard to many properties which reflect a difference in primary structure. These differences in properties result in the observed differences in combining constants and structural specificity. Even antibodies produced by individual inbred mice stimulated by the same antigen differ widely (Mattioli et al., 1968). Chemical differences observed for antibodies against a particular hapten include differences in amino acid compositions and differences in mutual combining regions holding together the H and L chains (Roholt et al., 1965a and 1965b). For example, differences in composition of the combining sites for a hapten have been shown by the fact that, for antibodies against a particular negatively charged hapten, the positive charge present in the site is due to the guanidinium group in some cases and the ammonium group in others (Freedman et al., 1968a). Also, differences exist in the tyrosine-containing peptides isolated from the sites (Roholt and Pressman, 1968), in the affinity-labeling pattern of the antibodies (Singer and Doolittle, 1966; Koyama et al., 1968a), in the hydrophobic character of the sites (Parker et al., 1967a and 1967b; Yoo and Parker, 1968), in the proximity of tryptophan (Little and Eisen, 1967), and in conformational changes brought about by iodination (Koyama et al., 1968b).

CHEMICAL NATURE OF COMBINING SITES OF ANTIBODY MOLECULES

Much information has recently been obtained about the chemical nature of the combining regions of antibody molecules, i.e., the contact amino acids in the combining region. Nearly all such information has been obtained by the use of antibodies directed against simple haptens, such as those Landsteiner and his colleagues employed so effectively in laying foundations for structure-activity relationships.

Most of this information has been obtained from studies of the effect of chemical alteration of antibody on its activity (Pressman and Grossberg, 1968, Chap.·5). Such studies are carried out by treating antibody with a reagent that is known to react with a particular chemical group. Loss of activity is indicative of an effect on the binding site. However, care must be used in interpreting such loss of activity. Even if the antibody is inactivated by reaction with a particular reagent, it must be proven that the loss of activity is caused by a reaction in the binding site and not by a chemical alteration of the general structure of the protein elsewhere in the antibody molecule. Such proof has been obtained in many cases. Furthermore, many reagents which are considered to react only with certain groups of amino acid residues do in fact react to some degree with other residues. Therefore, it is important to demonstrate just which type of residue is attacked and to relate the attack of the particular residue to the loss of antibody activity.

In determining whether a chemical reaction has affected the binding site of antibody and whether certain amino acid residues are present in the site, use is made of the following criteria: (1) There is a loss of binding activity as measured by equilibrium dialysis. A loss of precipitating activity is not conclusive because the chemical alteration could affect precipitation of antibody without affecting the site. (2) The binding activity is recovered upon reversal of the chemical alteration. (3) The presence of hapten during the chemical reaction protects the site against inactivation. (4) The amino acid residue affected is isolated and identified as coming from the site; for example, by the paired-label technique (Pressman and Grossberg, 1968, p. 182).

Although loss of activity on chemical alteration and protection of activity by the presence of hapten against such loss strongly implies a reaction in the site, the possibility remains that the effective reaction takes place elsewhere on the molecule, stabilizing a conformation of the molecule in which the binding site is altered. However, it would then be necessary for the presence of hapten in the site to stabilize a conformation in which the reactivity of this key residue is reduced (Pressman and Grossberg, 1968, p. 172). This indirect mechanism is unlikely on the basis of much of the present evidence.

Most of the information about the chemical composition of antibody sites has been obtained with four different antibodies: those directed against the p-azobenzenearsonate group (anti-R_p antibody), the p-azobenzoate group (anti-X_p antibody), the 3-azopyridine group (anti-P_3 antibody), and the p-azophenyltrimethylammonium group (anti-A_p antibody). Information is thus available about antibodies against two negative groups, a neutral group, and a positively charged group.

A summary of the groups present in these antibody sites, as indicated by the chemical modifications so far carried out, is given in Table 1.

A *negatively charged group* is present in the combining sites of antibodies directed against the positively charged group (anti-A_p antibodies). The negatively charged group is a carboxylate (Grossberg and Pressman, 1960). The other antibodies studied do not have a carboxylate in the site.

A *positively charged group* is present in the combining sites of anti-

TABLE 1

Groups Implicated as Being in the Antibody Site
(Rabbit Antibody)

	Anti-R_p $(AsO_3^=)$	Anti-X_p (COO^-)	Anti-P_3 (Pyridine)	Anti-A_p $N(CH_3)_3^+$
CHARGE				
Ion effects		+		+
Hapten		+		+
CARBOXYLATE				
Esterification	−	−	−	+
Reversal				+
pH 4				+
AMINO				
Maleylation	+	+	−	−
Reversal	+	+		
Polyalanylation	+	(?)*	−	−
Acetylation (low level)	+	+NP†	−	−
Carbamylation	+	+NP†		−
Carboxymethylation	+	(?)*		−
Amidination	+			
GUANIDINIUM				
Butanedione	+	+	−	−
Glyoxal	+	+	−	−
HYDROXYL				
Acetylation	+	+	+	+
Reversal	+	+	+	+
TYROSINE				
Iodination	+	+	+	+
Diazonium coupling	+	+		+
pH	+	+	+	+
Paired label	+	+		
TRYPTOPHAN	In sites of anti di- and tri-nitrophenyl antibody indicated by spectral shift of bound ligand			
HYDROPHOBIC RESIDUES	In sites of some antibodies indicated by enhancement of fluorescence of bound ligand			

*(?) = very small effect
†NP = no protection by ligand against loss of activity

bodies against negative charges (anti-X_p and anti-R_p antibodies). In some antibody molecules the positive group is guanidinium (Freedman et al., 1968a; Grossberg and Pressman, 1968). In others it appears to be ammonium (Freedman et al., 1968b and 1968c). Suggestive evidence for the presence of histidine in sites has been obtained for some anti-R_p preparations (Koyama et al., 1968a). In the case of anti-R_p antibodies, it has been possible to separate the molecules with ammonium in the site from those with guanidinium in the site (Freedman et al., 1968a).

The presence of an *amino group* is implicated in some anti-R_p antibody sites by maleylation, polyalanylation, carbamylation, carboxymethylation, amidination, and a low level of acetylation (Pressman and Grossberg, 1968; Freedman et al., 1968b and 1968c). The anti-X_p antibody shows loss of binding activity by maleylation, acetylation, and carboxymethylation. However, in some instances it is not certain that an amino group was present in the anti-X_p site because protection could not be achieved. The particular reactions used to alter amino groups have no effect on anti-P_3 or anti-A_p antibodies.

Guanidinium contributes the positive charge present in the sites of much anti-R_p and anti-X_p antibody (Freedman et al., 1968a; Grossberg and Pressman, 1968).

A *hydroxyl group* is present in the sites of all four antibodies, as shown by acetylation and reversal of the acetylation reaction (Pressman and Grossberg, 1968, p. 191). This hydroxyl group appears to be that of a *tyrosine,* indicated by the effect of the iodination reaction for all four antibodies (Pressman and Grossberg, 1968, p. 174), the effect of diazonium coupling for those tested (Pressman and Grossberg, 1968, p. 198), and the isolation of a tyrosine from the sites of anti-R_p and anti-X_p antibodies by the paired-label technique (Pressman and Grossberg, 1968, p. 182; Roholt and Pressman, 1968). The presence of tyrosine in sites is also implied by the decrease in binding at high pH values. A tyrosine group appears to be present in the combining sites of nearly all the antibodies investigated by the authors. However, Koshland et al. (1965) have found no evidence for its presence in one pool of anti-A_p antibody.

Other types of evidence have contributed information on the composition of antibody sites. The presence of *hydrophobic amino acid residues* is made apparent in the sites of certain antibodies when these antibodies combine with particular ligands. The combination results in enhancement of fluorescence of the ligand due to the change in environment. This is the case with antibodies against the 1, 4- and 1, 8-azonaphthalenesulfonate groups and the 1, 5-dimethylaminonaphthalenesulfonyl group (Parker et al., 1967a and 1967b; Yoo and Parker, 1968; Winkler, 1962; Yoo et al., 1967). These effects correlate with those observed when the ligands are transferred from aqueous to nonpolar media.

Tryptophan appears to be situated in the sites of antibodies directed against the dinitro- and trinitrobenzene groups, as Little and Eisen (1967) have deduced from spectral evidence of complex formation between ligand and tryptophan residues of antibodies. Quenching of fluorescence of the antibody when it binds ligand has been interpreted to indicate the presence of tryptophan near the site (Velick et al., 1960). The evidence cited above for the presence of groups in the site does not mean that the combining sites of all antibodies directed toward the particular hapten contain that group. It has indeed been observed in some cases that only some of the molecules contained a particular residue in the site (Freedman et al., 1968a). The activity of the remaining molecules was not affected by the chemical alteration even though in these molecules all of the particular residues had been altered. It would be very interesting to isolate the unaffected molecules following chemical alteration and see if they are free of molecules containing that residue in the site.

LIMITED HETEROGENEITY OF ANTIBODIES

It does not appear, as has been previously assumed, that the IgG antibodies produced by an individual animal represent a continuously heterogeneous population, composed of antibodies with binding constants following a Gaussian distribution. On the contrary, it does appear that only a few molecular species of antibody make up the bulk of antibody produced in each individual animal.

A mechanism for the latter situation has been proposed. In a given individual animal, of the many different cells which can produce IgG antibody capable of reacting with the particular hapten, only a few cells are stimulated to produce antibody. Each one of these cells multiplies and produces antibody molecules of only a particular structure. The other cells do not multiply and are repressed in their capacity to make antibodies reacting with this hapten. Thus the antibody produced in the individual animals can have markedly different characteristics, entirely on a chance basis, depending on which particular cells are stimulated. This mechanism would explain the large differences in the properties of antibodies produced in an individual animal. It should be pointed out that, until recently, the binding data for antibodies have been considered on the basis that a completely continuous heterogeneous population is present, and average binding constants and a heterogeneity coefficient have been calculated on that basis. However, curves very close to those of the experimental curves can be obtained on the consideration that only a few different species of antibodies are present, though with different binding constants (Roholt et al., 1968). When plotted by the usual methods this latter consideration gives binding curves and constants very similar to those obtained previously.

Many of the differences found in antisera from different individuals would not be observed unless the antibody from each were predominantly composed of a homogeneous population of molecules, or at least a few homogeneous populations.

Marked differences in combining constants for antibodies formed in response to a particular antigen in a single strain of mice (Mattioli et al., 1968) would not be observed unless a limited heterogeneity was the rule.

It has been found (Roholt and Pressman, 1968) that peptides which have been isolated from the site and which contain a tyrosine have different amino acid sequences for antibodies from different individual rabbits. In order to observe such a peptide, it would be necessary for an appreciable fraction of all the molecules in the population to have the particular sequence in their sites. If there were a continuous heterogeneity, the peptide from the site would necessarily come from the conservative region of the molecule. Otherwise, the quantity of peptide would not be great enough for detection. That this is not the case is shown by the isolation of different peptides from different individuals (Roholt and Pressman, 1968).

The variance in the effect of a particular reagent on different pools of antibodies from individual rabbits also indicates a similar limited heterogeneity for the individual pools (Roholt and Pressman, 1968; Koyama et al., 1968a and 1968b). Differences observed in affinity-labeling properties also indicate a limited heterogeneity, since the reactivity of the residues available for labeling varies from animal to animal (Singer and Doolittle, 1966; Koyama et al., 1968a).

It has been shown (Roholt et al., 1965a and 1965b; Edelman et al., 1963; Franek and Nezlin, 1963) that when antibody molecules are dissociated into light and heavy chains and are separated, the chains reassociate with a degree of specificity such that those chains which combine to give good antibody molecules are preferentially combined. For such chains to recombine correctly, there must be appreciable amounts of the same type of antibody molecule, i.e., the origin of the chains must be a population of molecules of limited heterogeneity.

The effect of iodination in causing conformational changes and alteration in the affinity-labeling characteristics, which differ for antibodies from individual animals (Koyama et al., 1968b), again points very strongly toward distinct characteristics for the antibodies from individual animals.

On one occasion, as reported by Nisonoff et al. (1967), the population of antibody molecules was sufficiently homogeneous to permit crystallization. In other instances, heterogeneity has been observed to be limited. Thus, in particular pools of antibodies, investigators have obtained anti-hapten antibodies whose light chains migrate as a single band on disc electrophoresis (Roholt et al., 1968; Brenneman and Singer,

1968). This requires that all the light chains be of a single charge class. In one of these cases two bands were observed with light chains from the antibodies formed during one six month period, whereas for light chains from antibodies formed in a subsequent period only one band was seen. This means that light chains of only two charged types were formed initially and subsequently all light chains of one of these charged types were discontinued. This observation is most easily explained by a model of limited heterogeneity.

In all of these instances, a given individual appears to be producing predominantly a few types of antibody molecules, each of which differs significantly from those produced by another individual.

SOME STRUCTURAL CONSIDERATIONS OF ANTIBODY-HAPTEN COMBINATION

It is interesting to consider which parts of a specific hapten group contribute to the combination of the hapten with antibody. Much work has been done to determine the effect of changing or "omitting" various substituents on a particular structure on a benzene ring, for example, and to determine the residual reactivity. These experiments lead to considerations of just what structures are important for a particular combination. For instance, in antibody to the *p*-azobenzoate ion, what are the important structures to be considered? The carboxylate group is very important, since replacing it by hydrogen to give azobenzene results in essentially no combination. Likewise, replacing the benzene ring by either a hydrogen or a methyl to give formate or acetate results in essentially no combination. Replacement of the carboxylate by a structurally similar group, the nitro group, results in essentially no combination. Thus the nitro group does not compensate for the carboxylate, presumably due largely to lack of negative charge. In addition there may be other structural differences, such as differences in degree of hydration of the carboxylate and nitro groups, which are not readily apparent, but which may be of great importance.

Next it is of interest to consider what happens when the structure under consideration has two obviously important groups, such as the carboxyl groups in the 5-azoisophthalate ion (Pressman and Grossberg, 1968, p. 95). It might be expected that replacement of one of the groups by the easily accommodated hydrogen group would still lead to appreciable combination with antibody, since one carboxylate is still retained. However, with the replacement of the group by hydrogen a very large part of the interaction energy is lost. Replacement with a nitro group is not very effective since metanitrobenzoate does not combine well either. Thus, for adequate combination of a hapten with this antibody both carboxylate groups are required. In the antibenzoate system however, where a single carboxylate is the determinant, a single carboxylate on the hapten is sufficient to hold the antibody and hapten together.

Similarly in the anti-3,5-dinitroazobenzene system (Pressman and Grossberg, 1968, p. 105) both nitro groups are required for combination, whereas in the anti-*p*-nitroazobenzene system (Pressman and Grossberg, 1968, p. 65) only one is required. Again in the anti-3-nitro-5-carboxy-azobenzene system (Pressman and Grossberg, 1968, p. 111) both the nitro and the carboxyl groups in the correct positions are required since neither group alone, as in nitrobenzene or benzoate, is sufficient to hold the hapten and antibody together. Thus it appears that a certain energy combination is required to hold antigen and antibody together and this energy is derived from the various component parts.

In the case of antibodies against the steroids, the various structural components and the steric configuration of the molecule play a very important role. It would appear that the A ring is significant in determining the lack of cross-reaction of anti-estradiol antibodies with testosterone. The antibody directed against the estradiol is directed against the planar benzene ring and thus does not seem to be able to accommodate the puckered saturated ring of testosterone or androsterone. The angular methyl groups, phenolic and aliphatic hydroxyls, and the ketone group are probably important determinative structures also. The nonpolar character of most steroid molecules is probably of major importance also.

In conclusion, from the practical point of view, we would like to state that antibodies reactive with an individual steroid nucleus will be of many different primary amino acid sequences and directed individually against different structural features or combinations of structural features. Thus individual antisera will have antibody populations of greater importance for certain assays than other assays.

REFERENCES

Brenneman, L., and S. J. Singer. 1968. The generation of antihapten antibodies with electrophoretically homogeneous L chains. Proc. Nat. Acad. Sci. USA, 60:258–264.

Edelman, G. M., D. E. Olins, J. A. Gally, and N. D. Zinder. 1963. Reconstitution of immunologic activity by interaction of polypeptide chains of antibodies. Proc. Nat. Acad. Sci. USA, 50:753–761.

Franek, F., and R. S. Nezlin. 1963. The role of different peptide chains of antibody in the antigen-antibody reaction. Biokhimiia, 28:193–203.

Freedman, M. H., A. L. Grossberg, and D. Pressman. 1968a. Evidence for ammonium and guanidinium groups in the combining sites of anti-*p*-azobenzenearsonate antibodies—separation of two different populations of antibody molecules. J. Biol. Chem., 243:6186–6195.

———A. L. Grossberg, and D. Pressman. 1968b. The effects of complete modification of amino groups on the antibody activity of antihapten antibodies. Reversible inactivation with maleic anhydride. Biochemistry (Wash.), 7:1941–1950.

————A. L. Grossberg, and D. Pressman. 1968c. Participation of amino groups in the active sites of antibodies. Immunochemistry, 5:367–381.

Grossberg, A. L., and D. Pressman. 1960. Nature of the combining site of antibody against a hapten bearing a positive charge. J. Amer. Chem. Soc., 82:5478–5482.

————and D. Pressman. 1968. Modification of arginine in the active sites of antibodies. Biochemistry (Wash.), 7:272–279.

Koshland, M. E., F. M. Englberger, and S. M. Gaddone. 1965. Evidence against the universality of a tyrosyl residue at antibody combining sites. Immunochemistry, 2:115–125.

Koyama, J., A. L. Grossberg, and D. Pressman. 1968a. Variability among anti-*p*-azobenzenearsonate antibody preparations as revealed by affinity labeling. Biochemistry (Wash.), 7:1935–1940.

———— A. L. Grossberg, and D. Pressman. 1968b. Conformational changes in anti-*p*-azobenzenearsonate antibody caused by iodination. Biochemistry (Wash.), 7:2369–2375.

Little, E. R., and H. N. Eisen. 1967. Evidence for tryptophan in the active sites of antibodies to polynitrobenzenes. Biochemistry (Wash.), 6:3119–3125.

Mattioli, C. A., Y. Yagi, and D. Pressman. 1968. Production and properties of mouse antihapten antibodies. J. Immun., 101:939–948.

Nisonoff, A., S. Zappacosta, and R. Jureziz. 1967. Properties of crystallized rabbit anti-*p*-azobenzoate antibody. Cold Spring Harbor Symp. Quant. Biol., 32:89–93.

Parker, C. W., T.-J. Yoo, M. C. Johnson, and S. M. Godt. 1967a. Fluorescent probes for the study of the antibody-hapten reaction. I. Binding of the 5-dimethylaminonaphthalene-1-sulfonamido group by homologous rabbit antibody. Biochemistry (Wash.), 6:3408–3416.

———— S. M. Godt, and M. C. Johnson. 1967b. Fluorescent probes for the study of the antibody-hapten reaction. II. Variation in the antibody combining site during the immune response. Biochemistry (Wash.), 6:3417–3427.

Pressman, D., and A. L. Grossberg. 1968. The Structural Basis of Antibody Specificity. New York, W. A. Benjamin, Inc.

Roholt, O. A., A. L. Grossberg, and D. Pressman. 1968. Limited heterogeneity of antibodies. Fed. Proc., 27:684.

———— and D. Pressman. 1968. Structural differences between antibodies against the same hapten by individual rabbits. Immunochemistry, 5:265–275.

———— G. Radzimski, and D. Pressman. 1965a. Preferential recombination of antibody chains to form effective binding sites. J. Exp. Med., 122:785–798.

———— G. Radzimski, and D. Pressman. 1965b. Polypeptide chains of antibody: Effective binding sites require specificity in combination. Science, 147:613–615.

Singer, S. J., and R. F. Doolittle. 1966. Antibody active sites and immuno-globulin molecules. Science, 153:13–24.

Velick, S. F., C. W. Parker, and H. N. Eisen. 1960. Excitation energy transfer and the quantitative study of the antibody hapten reaction. Proc. Nat. Acad. Sci. USA, 46:1470–1482.

Winkler, M. H. 1962. A molecular probe for the antibody site. J. Molec. Biol., 4:118–120.

Yoo, T.-J., and C. W. Parker. 1968. Fluorescent enhancement in anti-body-hapten interaction 1-anilinonaphthalene-8-sulfonate as a fluorescent molecular probe for anti-azonaphthalene sulfonate antibody. Immunochemistry, 5:143–153.

——— O. A. Roholt, and D. Pressman. 1967. Specific binding activity of isolated light chains of antibodies. Science, 157:707–709.

DISCUSSION

B. V. CALDWELL.   Would you comment on whether or not limited heterogeneity might be modified by repeated immunizations or whether it is better to immunize for a short period of time and take repeated bleedings.

D. PRESSMAN.   I think that as immunization proceeds the antibodies become less and less heterogeneous. Styles change in the ways of preparing antibodies. People thought that it was quite necessary to use early sera because they would get the least degree of cross-reactivity. I think that as one injects more and more, one finds that particular clones of cells start to predominate and the antibodies become more and more homogeneous. As animals get older, their globulin picture simplifies greatly, or if animals are irradiated, their globulin picture also becomes simpler. It seems that particular clones of cells survive and old animals will show spikes of globulin which look quite a bit like myeloma proteins in their homogeneity. I think the same situation pertains with antibodies, in that there is a predominance of particular cell clones which persist and yield a quite homogeneous antibody. The animals that we have studied were always injected for a long time because of the types of experiments we were carrying out. Indeed, Dr. Roholt has been able to show that the antibodies produced in certain rabbits are simple after long injections, in that a good number of animals showed one or two bands in their light chain. Of course this means an increased homogeneity.

A. MUNCK.   Dr. Pressman, would you say something about the applicability of the labeling and iodination of steroid-antibody complexes? Do such reactions go at low temperatures, 4°C, for example? I also have in mind the usefulness of such methods in the study of steroid hormone receptor complexes, which may dissociate quite rapidly even at room temperature.

D. PRESSMAN.   I think the best method for labeling the receptor molecule or site is the affinity-labeling method, using a steroid with a chemically reactive group. The steroid would bind with the receptor site, and then just tie itself in. This kind of reaction has been used by Bernard Baker who tries to inhibit particular enzymes by feeding the enzyme substrate with reactive groups which hold the substrate in the site. He has been quite successful with these methods.

S. Lieberman.   Could you please elaborate upon the enhanced fluorescence the hapten exhibits when it is absorbed on the antibody? To what is this phenomenon due?

D. Pressman.   All fluorescent substances absorb light of one wavelength and give off light of a different wavelength. These particular sulfonic acids have the property of exhibiting little fluorescence unless they are in a nonpolar environment. If you take this anilinonaphthalene sulfonic acid and measure its fluorescence in aqueous medium it is practically nonfluorescent. If you put it in ethyl alcohol, you will find increasing fluorescence with increasing concentrations of alcohol. If you put it into alcohols which are less polar than ethanol, you find that it fluoresces still more. There are also other effects which enhance fluorescence. However, the greatest effect is the nonpolar effect. When the molecule combines with the antibody site, the increase in fluorescence is attributed to the nonpolar character of the site. Actually there is a whole field of chemistry using these fluorescent molecules as probes to determine nonpolar regions in molecules.

G. Barnes.   Dr. Pressman, I wonder if there is any evidence that certain cell types might be involved in the heterogeneity picture. Do you know of any work where people have actually labeled particular cell types according to their specific antibody type?

D. Pressman.   Well, there is work now going on to look for receptor sites on lymphoid cells to determine which cells bind particular antigens or haptens.

A. Sehon.   Since one would expect that the male should be more tolerant to testosterone and the female more tolerant to estrogenic protein derivatives, I would like to know if others have determined whether there is any relationship between the sex of the animals and their response to particular protein-steroid conjugates.

D. Pressman.   I guess this should really be answered by the audience since we have a large body of individuals who could share their experiences.

S. Gross.   We have done this. Our female rabbits were less successful. Their quantitative precipitin antibody titers were lower than those of male rabbits. It is likely that soluble complexes are formed in the females.

D. Bullock.   I can support Dr. Gross' observation that male rabbits seem to produce higher antibody titers against estradiol conjugates than do females, although this also is an impression based on few animals. Presumably, endogenous estrogen in the female lowers the antibody titer and ovariectomized females should do as well as males. I wonder if Dr. Gross or others have found this to be so?

S. Gross.   We have not studied the biologic effects of estradiol antibodies.

N. Jiang.   We have some experience with immunizing both male and female rabbits with estradiol and estrone derivatives. We have four rabbits per group. We find there is no difference in the immunoresponsiveness in the male and the female rabbits.

K. Werder.   I have a question concerning radioiodination of the antibody. Is it a consistent result that all binding sites of the antibody are destroyed by the iodination procedure? This has some importance for the immunoradiometric assay of peptide hormones (Miles and Hales, 1968. *Nature* 219: 186) where one wants to iodinate the antibodies instead of the antigen (regular immunoassay) and to be sure that all binding sites are destroyed except one, which is protected by binding to the immunoadsorbent.

D. Pressman.   In general, the antibodies are not affected in specificity by low levels of iodination. However, at higher levels, sites are nearly always hit. Occasionally we have an antibody preparation which can be iodinated without affecting the site.

A. Grossberg.   I think the question was whether iodination would necessarily destroy the site. It should be realized that sites are hit only at quite high levels of iodine incorporation whereas trace labeling with iodine can be done with only one or fewer iodine atoms per molecule. Thus, one can easily trace-label antibody molecules with iodine without any loss of activity.

S. Gross.   Miles reported iodination of insulin antibodies after binding with hapten coupled to a solid matrix. Acid elution recovered labeled antibodies whose binding sites had been protected by hapten.

G. Richardson.   I wonder if anyone has employed the property of acquired biologic tolerance, that is, making an animal tolerant to a hapten in the intrauterine or neonatal phase. This might eliminate the haptens you do not want to measure with an immunoassay. The animal could be immunized later on with the steroid hapten you do want to measure.

D. Pressman.   There have been a good many experiments concerned with this particular aspect, but I do not think we have time to go into them now.

2

EARLY APPROACHES TO PRODUCTION, ANALYSIS, AND USE OF STEROID-SPECIFIC ANTISERA

Lawrence Goodfriend

The Harry Webster Thorp Laboratories,
Division of Immunochemistry and Allergy, McGill University Clinic,
Royal Victoria Hospital, Montreal, Canada

Alec Sehon

Department of Immunology, University of Manitoba
Winnipeg, Canada

INTRODUCTION

We feel compelled to begin this presentation on a rather personal note. It is now a decade since we carried out studies on the antigenicity of estrone-protein conjugates, studies which neither of us, probably to our regret, continued subsequently (Goodfriend and Sehon, 1958, 1960, 1961a, 1961b; Goodfriend et al., 1961). Ten years is a rather long time for a study to lie dormant in one's head, and unfortunately no new data are produced with increase in time of this kind of incubation! While we feel flattered to have been asked to participate in this meeting in spite of these circumstances, because of them we shall have to circumscribe our contribution within the narrow limits of an historic summary of these early experiments. Nevertheless, we shall try to improve matters by referring as frequently as possible to the extensive and very beautiful investigations of an array of steroid-protein conjugates, which were concurrently and independently carried out by Dr. Lieberman and his associates at Columbia University (Erlanger et al., 1957, 1959; Beiser et al., 1959; Lieberman et al., 1959). We would like to stress here how very aware we are of the fact that the work of the Columbia group has been largely instrumental in stimulating the proliferation of studies on steroid-specific antibodies, as witness the proceedings of this symposium.

The full potential value of studies with steroid-specific antisera was only vaguely sensed when we began our studies. What particularly impressed us at that time was the considerable body of clinical reports which suggested the possibility that steroid-specific antibodies were the etiologic factors in premenstrual disorders of an allergic nature (for review, see Vallery-Radot, 1957). Such antibodies could conceivably arise as an immunopathologic response to endogenous or exogenously administered steroids following their conjugation with macromolecules of the host, such as serum proteins.

The immediate objective of our studies was to establish whether or not steroids could indeed act as haptens (Landsteiner, 1945). That is, whether or not steroid-specific antibodies could be elicited (in rabbits) by immunization with steroid-protein conjugates. Continuing the work begun by Landsteiner, numerous low-molecular-weight chemicals had been coupled to proteins and the resulting conjugates shown to stimulate the production of anti-hapten antibodies as well as antibodies to the carrier proteins. The question posed in our studies, and in the studies of the Columbia group, was whether by the same methodologic approach antibodies could be elicited to steroids, which could be considered as prototypes of low-molecular-weight chemicals indigenous to the host. This may seem like a trite question today, but it must be remembered that at the time of our studies only two instances of the successful preparation of antisera to low-molecular-weight metabolites were known, that of Clutton et al. (1938) to thyroxine, and Sheldon et al. (1941) to histamine. Furthermore, Mooser and Grilichess (1941) had reported that their androstenediol-protein conjugates failed to elicit rabbit antibodies to the steroid moieties. Consequently, the outcome of our studies was by no means certain. In addition to providing yet another demonstration of antibodies to low-molecular-weight metabolites, a positive outcome would, we anticipated, make available reagents for investigation of endocrinologic problems such as those discussed by Dr. Lieberman, including the problem of immunoassay of steroids. The latter investigations naturally had to await the decisive demonstration by immunochemical methods of the steroid specificity of antisera to steroid-protein conjugates.

PREPARATION AND PROPERTIES OF STEROID-PROTEIN CONJUGATES

With the aforementioned motivating influences at work, both we and the Columbia group proceeded in the latter 1950's to couple steroids to proteins by stable covalent linkages. The emphasis is on stable here,

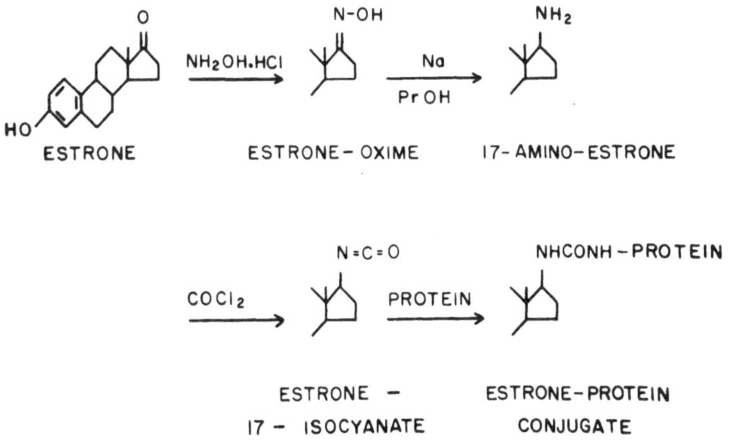

Fig. 1. Flowsheet for preparation of estrone-17-carbamido-protein conjugates. *From* Goodfriend and Sehon. 1958. *Can. J. Biochem. Physiol.,* 36:1178. Reproduced by permission of the National Research Council of Canada.

because of the instructive failure by Mooser and Grilichess (1941) to obtain antibodies to androstenediol, probably owing to the easily hydrolyzable ester linkages by which these workers bound the steroid to the immunizing carrier protein.

In our studies, we coupled estrone to proteins via highly stable carbamido-linkages at the C-17 and C-2 positions (Goodfriend and Sehon, 1958; Goodfriend et al., 1961). To prepare C-17-estronyl conjugates, we synthesized estrone-17-isocyanate (Fig. 1) and coupled it separately to HSA,* BSA, RSA and to OA; the reaction occurring primarily with the ε-NH$_2$ group of protein lysine. Estrone-2-carbamido conjugates were prepared by coupling the 2-isocyanate derivative to HSA and BSA (Fig. 2).

Whereas in our studies, a single steroid, estrone, was coupled to a number of carrier proteins of different antigenic specificities, the Columbia group conjugated a variety of steroids via amide linkages to a single protein carrier, BSA, using elegant techniques of wide applicability (Erlanger et al., 1957, 1959). The essence of their methods is shown in Figure 3. The Schotten-Baumann reaction was employed to couple testosterone to BSA: the C-17 hydroxyl of the steroid was converted to the acyl-chloride which could react with ε-amino groups of the lysine residues. Most of the conjugates were prepared by reacting BSA with mixed anhydrides formed between iso-butylchlorocarbonate and carboxylate

* HSA, BSA, RSA=human, bovine, and rabbit serum albumin, respectively; OA= chicken ovalbumin.

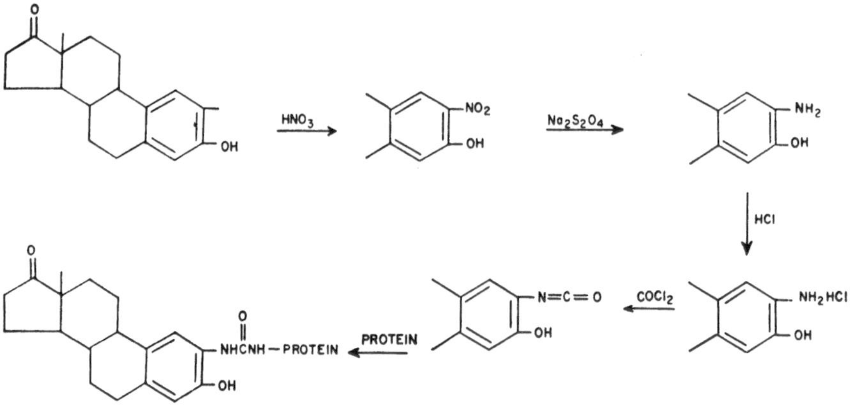

Fig. 2. Flowsheet for preparation of estrone-2-carbamido-protein conjugates. *From* Goodfriend et al. 1961. *Can. J. Biochem. Physiol.,* 39:968. Reproduced by permission of the National Research Council of Canada.

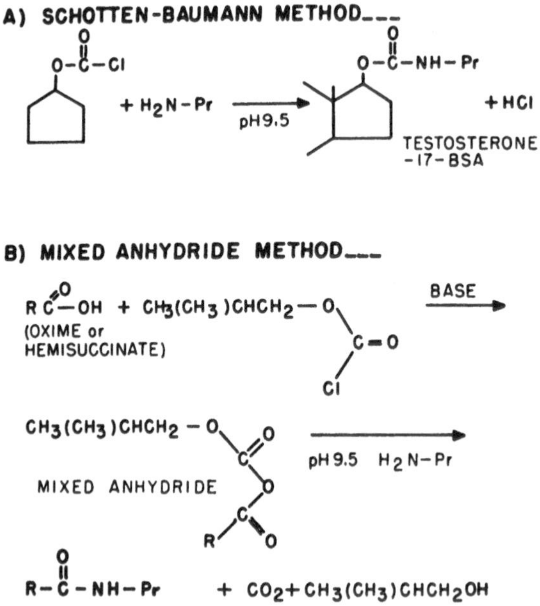

A) SCHOTTEN-BAUMANN METHOD.___

TESTOSTERONE -17-BSA

B) MIXED ANHYDRIDE METHOD.___

Fig. 3. Methods employed for coupling of steroid derivatives to protein. Pr = protein residue. *From* Lieberman et al. 1959. *Recent Progr. Hormone Res.,* 15:168.

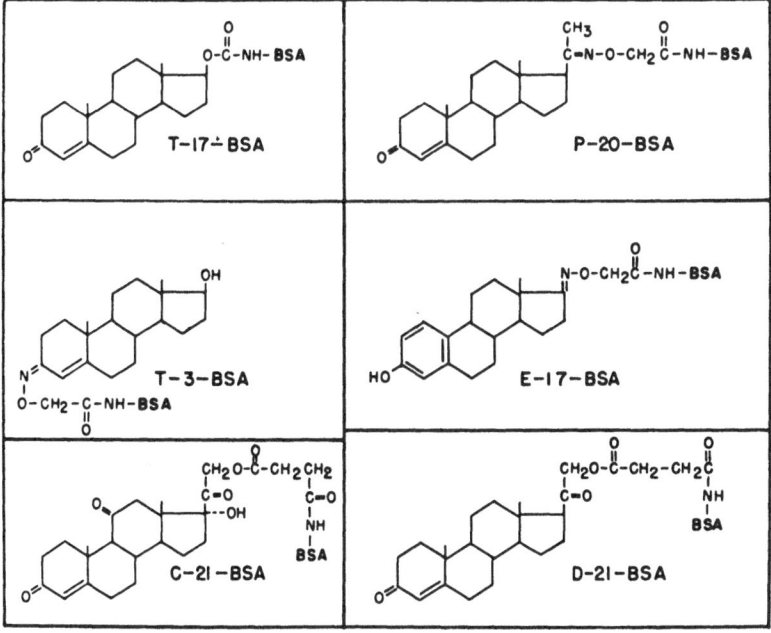

Fig. 4. Six steroid hormone-bovine serum albumin conjugates and their designations. *From* Lieberman et al. 1959. *Recent Progr. Hormone Res.*, 15:170.

oxime or succinate steroid derivatives, reaction occurring with protein lysine. The conjugates shown in Figure 4, which were prepared with testosterone, progesterone, estrone, cortisone, and deoxycorticosterone, serve to emphasize that the Columbia group developed the methodology for coupling a broad spectrum of steroids with minimal perturbation of the native steroid configurations.

After purification, the steroid-protein conjugates were characterized chemically in a number of ways (Goodfriend and Sehon, 1958, 1961a; Goodfriend et al., 1961; Erlanger et al., 1957, 1959). We have stated that the reactive functions grafted onto the steroids reacted primarily with the ε-amino groups of protein lysine. This was shown by both groups of investigators from the results of free-amino and UV spectrophotometric assays. That some 20 to 30 steroid residues had been coupled per protein molecule was further confirmed by the Columbia group using a dinitrophenylation technique and in our studies by radioactive analysis of 16^{-14}C-tagged estronyl conjugates. As would be anticipated from transformation of the potentially cationic ε-amino groups of the lysine residues into relatively neutral functions, at near-neutral pH's, the conjugates had significantly greater anodic electrophoretic mobilities than the carrier proteins.

TABLE 1

Hapten Inhibition of Precipitation of Anti-C-2-EHSA Serum Absorbed with HSA[a]

	μg N precipitated		
C-2-EHSA added (μg N)	Uninhibited	Inhibited with 0.35 μmole of 2-amino-esterone	Inhibited with 1.24 μmoles of 2-nitro-estrone
5.125	39.0	13.0	6.0
10.25	68.0	19.5	10.0
20.5	85.0	17.0	10.5
41	73.5	11.0	8.0

[a]The antiserum was diluted four-fold with borate buffer (0.1 $\underline{M}$, pH 8.0). For the uninhibited and inhibited reactions, 2.0-ml volumes of buffer and steroid in buffer were added per tube, respectively. After Goodfriend et al. 1961. Can. J. Biochem. Physiol., 39:969. Reproduced by permission of the National Research Council of Canada.

ANALYSIS OF ANTISERA TO STEROID-PROTEIN CONJUGATES

We turn now to the specificity of rabbit antisera raised to the steroid-protein conjugates.

In our studies, rabbits were separately immunized with C-17- and C-2-EHSA* and the specificity of the antisera produced to each conjugate was established in cross-reaction and hapten-inhibition experiments. The results of these studies demonstrated the presence in the antisera of two major antibody populations: one with combining sites directed to the estronyl residues, the other to the protein moiety of the immunizing conjugates.

Some of the data obtained are summarized in the following:

(1) Using the quantitative precipitin technique, pooled antiserum to C-2-EHSA reacted with the immunizing conjugate, and, to a lesser extent, with HSA (Goodfriend et al., 1961). After quantitative removal of antibodies to HSA, the absorbed antiserum gave no reaction with α-naphthyl-carbamido-HSA, reacted only very slightly with C-17-EHSA (Goodfriend, 1960), but gave appreciable reaction with C-2-EHSA. The reaction with C-2-EHSA could be inhibited with 2-nitro- and 2-amino-estrone at micromole levels (Table 1). At these levels, the estrone derivatives were without effect on the precipitin reaction between HSA and the unabsorbed antiserum.

(2) The presence of two major antibody specificities in pooled antiserum to estrone-17-carbamido-HSA was revealed in experiments using the

* Estrone-17- and 2-carbamido human serum albumins, respectively.

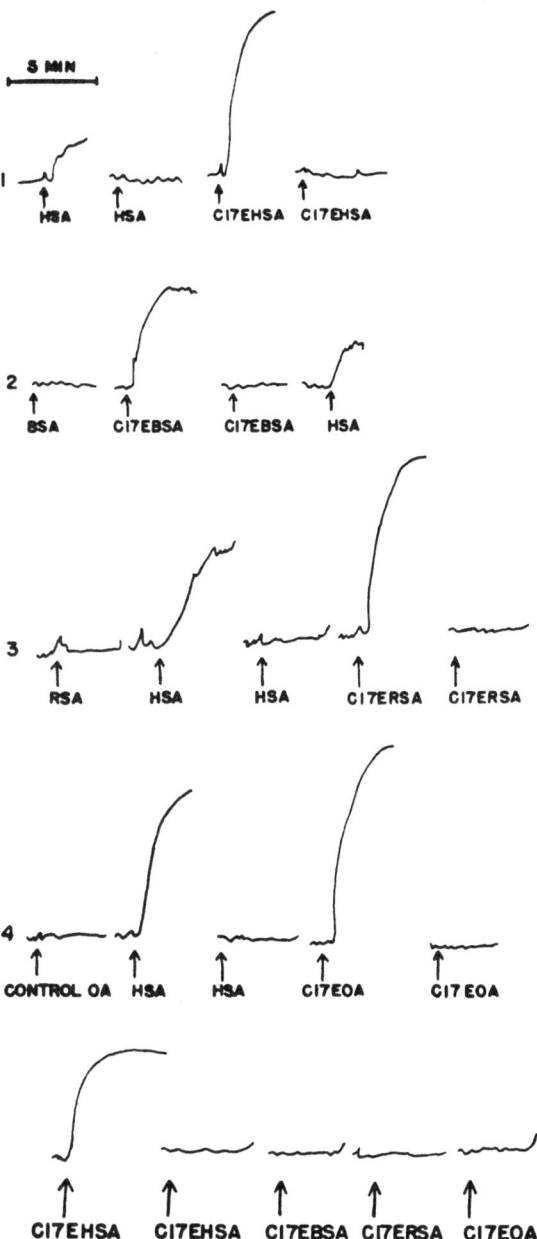

Fig. 5. In vitro anaphylaxis of guinea pig uteri passively sensitized with antiserum to C-17-EHSA on challenge with test antigens. *From* Goodfriend and Sehon. 1961a. *Can. J. Biochem. Physiol.*, 39:949. Reproduced by permission of the National Research Council of Canada.

quantitative precipitin and BDB-hemagglutination techniques, and more graphically by means of the Schultz-Dale technique (Goodfriend and Sehon, 1961a). In the latter studies, young female guinea pigs were passively sensitized by intraperitoneal injection of the rabbit antiserum to C-17-EHSA, their uteri excised, and segments mounted in the bath of a Schultz-Dale apparatus for reactivity to various test antigens.

As shown by the kymograph tracing in the uppermost part of Figure 5, addition of HSA to the bath elicited contraction of the sensitized uterine segments. Following desensitization to HSA, the addition of C-17-EHSA produced a further vigorous contraction. Except for HSA, none of the control proteins, BSA, RSA, OA, elicited contractions of the sensitized uteri. On the other hand, contractions were obtained with the C-17-estronyl conjugates formed with these proteins, a result in conformity with the presence of estrone-specific antibodies in the sensitizing antiserum.

(3) More definitive identification of estrone-specific antibodies in the

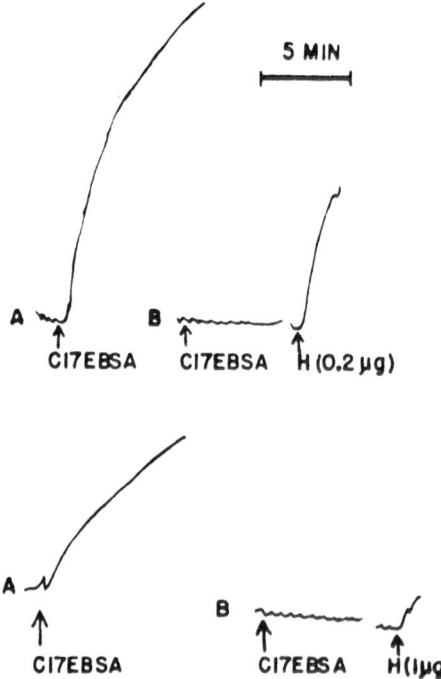

Fig. 6. Hapten inhibition of in vitro anaphylaxis. Guinea pig uterus passively sensitized with rabbit antiserum (1:4) to C-17-EHSA. Top: one uterine horn; bottom: other horn. A represents uninhibited reaction; B, the reaction after previous incubation of uterine segment with 2.0 μg/ml each of 17α-ethynyl estradiol-17ß (top) and estrone (bottom). *From* Goodfriend and Sehon. 1961a. *Can. J. Biochem. Physiol.*, 39:952. Reproduced by permission of the National Research Council of Canada.

"C-17 antiserum" was obtained by hapten inhibition of the Schultz-Dale reaction. In the uninhibited cases (Fig. 6) the uterine tissues sensitized with rabbit antiserum to C-17-EHSA contracted to C-17-EBSA and to HSA. However, prior incubation of uterine tissues from the same animals with 2 to 3 µg/ml of estrone or 17α-ethynyl-estradiol-17β (or estrone 17-carbamido-glycine) completely inhibited contraction to the heterologous C-17-estronyl conjugates but was without effect on the response to HSA. In contrast, levels of testosterone 17α-glucoside or 17α-hydroxycorticosterone of 50 to 100 µg/ml were ineffective in this system.

(4) The specificity of the antibodies to estrone was examined on a more quantitative basis using hapten inhibition of the turbidimetric reaction (Goodfriend and Sehon, 1961a). Parenthetically, to our knowledge these studies constituted the first use of the turbidimetric technique to demonstrate hapten specificity.

The upper curve of Figure 7 shows the time course of light scattered due to interaction of C-17-EBSA with antiserum to C-17-EHSA at optimum concentrations. The lower curves were obtained for the same reaction in the presence of 2 µg of estrone, 4 µg of 17α-ethynyl-estradiol-17β, and 5 µg of estrone-17-carbamido-glycine. Clearly, these steroids caused a substantial reduction in the amount of light scattered. While as little as

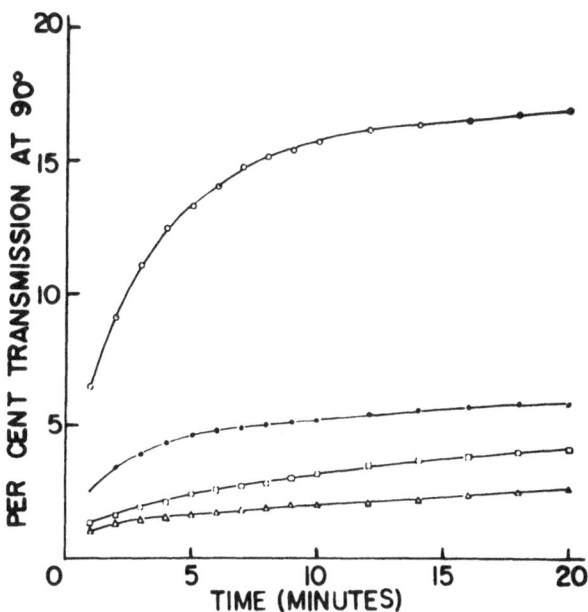

Fig. 7. Hapten inhibition of turbidity due to C-17-EBSA-anti-C-17-EHSA reaction: o = uninhibited, • = estrone (2 µg), Δ = 17α-ethynyl estradiol-17β (4 µg), and and □ = estrone-17-carbamido-glycine (5µg). *From* Goodfriend and Sehon. 1961a. *Can. J. Biochem. Physiol.,* 39:954. Reproduced by permission of the National Research Council of Canada.

TABLE 2

Hapten Inhibition of Turbidity Due to C-17-EBSA — Anti-C-17-EHSA Reaction

Test inhibitor	Amount added (μmoles)	% inhibition[a]
Estrone	0.007	66
Estrone-17-carbamido-glycine	0.013	85
Estrone-17-carbamido-glycine	0.026	99
17α-Ethynylestradiol-17β	0.013	76
17α-Ethynylestradiol-17β	0.026	89
17a-Hydroxycorticosterone-21-sodium succinate	0.44	31
Testosterone-17α-glucoside	0.44	76
2,6-Dimethyl-phenol	1.6	0
3,4-Dimethyl-phenol	1.6	16
(D,1)-Tyrosine	1.1	0

[a]Calculated on the basis of the turbidity readings at the 20-minute mark for the uninhibited and inhibited reactions. After Goodfriend and Sehon. 1961a. Can. J. Biochem. Physiol., 39:956. Reproduced by permission of the National Research Council of Canada.

10 to 20 mμmoles of estrone or the C-17-estronyl derivatives markedly suppressed the conjugate-anti-conjugate reaction (Table 2), such substances as tyrosine and the dimethylphenols showed little or no inhibitory activity at the 1000 mμmole level. On the other hand, appreciable inhibition was obtained with testosterone and corticosterone derivatives at the 400 to 500 mμmole level. Assuming little or no effect due to differences in C-17 side chains of these steroids, the relatively lower inhibitory capacity of the corticosterone compared to the testosterone derivatives may be interpreted as due to steric hindrance by the 11β-hydroxyl group at the antibody site. A similar reduction in inhibitory capacity due to the presence of an 11β-hydroxyl was found by the Columbia group for various steroid antibody systems, and we turn now to some of the results obtained in their study (Beiser et al., 1959; Lieberman et al., 1959).

Rabbit antisera prepared to various steroid-protein conjugates were found to contain precipitating antibodies to the immunizing carrier protein, BSA. After removal of these antibodies by absorption with BSA, the antisera were found still capable of precipitating with the conjugates. Hapten inhibition of the quantitative precipitin reaction, using various water soluble steroid derivatives as test inhibitors, demonstrated a high steroid specificity for the antibodies in the absorbed antisera. To illustrate, we cite two examples from their data.

(1) The results obtained with absorbed antiserum to cortisone-21-BSA are shown in Figure 8. The test inhibitors were employed at equal concentrations, and of these, cortisone succinate was most effective in inhibiting the precipitin reaction. It can be seen that the nature of the side chain at the C-17 position and of the function at the C-3 position were highly determinant with regard to specificity. The nature of the oxygen

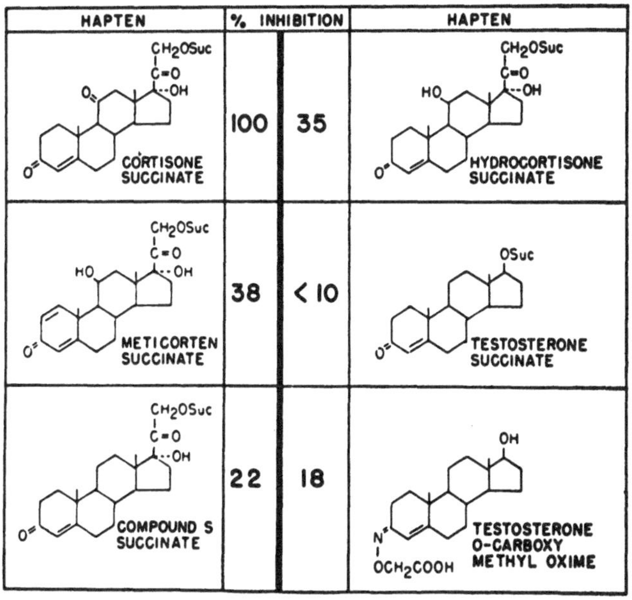

Fig. 8. Hapten inhibition test with anti-C-21-BSA. The data shown were obtained using all the haptens at the same concentration. *After* Lieberman et al. 1959. *Recent Progr. Hormone Res.*, 15:184.

function at C-11 was likewise of importance: replacement of the ketonic by the hydroxyl group reduced the extent of inhibition, while removal of the ketonic group, as in testosterone succinate, reduced this still further.

(2) Figure 9 shows the results obtained with antiserum to deoxy-corticosterone-21-BSA. Here too, test inhibitors with structures closely related to the immunizing hapten were most effective in inhibiting the precipitin reaction with BSA-absorbed antiserum. Three structural features of the immunizing hapten were apparently important in determining the antibody specificity: the α,β unsaturated carbonyl group in ring A, the nature of the oxygen function at C-11, and the nature of the side chain at C-17. As with the previous example, a β-hydroxyl function at C-11, as in hydrocortisone succinate, reduced the extent of inhibition while the presence of a C-11 ketonic group was without effect. The presence of a hydroxyl group at C-17, as in cortisone succinate, was without effect on the ability of the hapten to fit the antibody combining site. Aromatization of the A ring had a strong influence on inhibitory capacity. Nevertheless, the appreciable inhibitory activity obtained with estrone-17-O-carboxy-methyloxime demonstrated common stereochemical features for the estrone and corticosterone structures which enabled the latter to combine with the same antibody sites. Similarly, appreciable cross-reaction was reported for testosterone succinate with antibodies to estrone-17-O-carboxymethyloxime (Beiser et al., 1959).

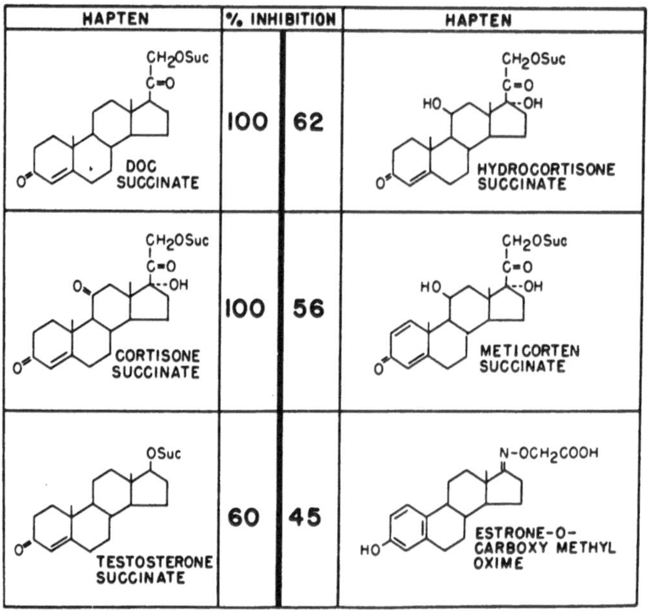

Fig. 9. Hapten inhibition test with anti-D-21-BSA. All the haptens were examined at the same concentration. *After* Lieberman et al. 1959. *Recent Progr. Hormone Res.,* 15:185.

Summarizing the results obtained by the Columbia group and in our own studies, we may say that the steroid residues of the conjugates funttioned haptenically in inducing steroid-specific antibodies. While each of the steroids coupled to protein gave rise to antibodies with structurally unique combining sites, they also led to the formation of antibodies able to cross-react with heterologous steroids. The extent of such cross-reaction depended on the nature of the A ring and on the presence or absence of substituents at certain positions of the steroid nucleus. The C-11 position appeared to have an important role, similar to that observed for Δ^4, 3-ketosteroid-albumin interaction (Westphal and Ashley, 1958).

SOME APPLICATIONS TO ENDOCRINOLOGIC PROBLEMS

With the preparation of steroid-specific antisera, reagents became available which could be applied to a variety of problems of endocrinologic interest. We shall now deal briefly with several of these.

Cellular Sites of Steroid Synthesis

As an example taken from our own studies on the potential use of steroid-specific antisera, we may cite our preliminary efforts to determine the cellular localization of estrogen in the rat ovary by the immuno-fluorescent technique (Goodfriend et al., 1961). Localization depends upon the formation of antigen-fluorescent antibody aggregates in sufficient amounts to make fluorescence discernible. This makes the detection of small, univalent molecules such as estrone or estradiol difficult, since the latter do not form precipitates with antibody. The possibility cannot be overlooked, however, that in some tissues steroid might be firmly fixed to cellular components in sufficiently high concentration for localization. We therefore attempted to localize estrogens in the rat ovary using fluorescein-labeled antibodies to C-2-EHSA.

Whereas ovarian slices derived from immature female rats showed no fluorescence on staining with the tagged antiserum, ovarian slices from untreated and FSH-stimulated mature rats showed green fluorescence in the cytoplasmic region of perifollicular cells (Fig. 10). In addition, we observed bright fluorescence of stroma cells throughout the ovaries of FSH-stimulated animals. While these results demonstrated the presence of some tissue component reacting with antibodies to the C-2-EHSA conjugate, further experiments would be required to determine if this component is identical with an estrogen-tissue complex. Such experiments would include, for example, specific inhibition of fluorescence by tagged antiserum to C-2-EHSA previously incubated with free estrone, and staining of mature ovaries throughout the entire estrous cycle. In spite of the incompleteness of this study, we were encouraged by it, in that the cells which took up the fluorescein-labeled antibodies to estrone-protein conjugate were thought, at least at the time of these studies, to be involved in the production of estrogens (Faleck, 1959).

Anti-Hormonal Activity of Steroid-Specific Antisera

In our own brief study relevant to this question (Goodfriend and Sehon, 1961b), we observed that mixtures of estrone and anti-estrone antiserum lacked estrogenic activity in the 6-hour uterotropic assay of Astwood (1938). As shown in Table 3, the addition of *normal* rabbit serum to estrone failed to suppress its estrogenic activity as measured by uterine to body weight ratios. In contrast, addition of estrone-specific rabbit antiserum completely abolished the uterotropic activity of the steroid.

More germane and extensive studies were done by the Columbia group, who reported that passive transfer of some of the steroid-specific antisera could indeed inhibit the hormonal activity of exogenously administered steroids (Lieberman et al., 1959). These observations were amplified and made more definitive in a subsequent study (Neri et al., 1964). This study showed that passive administration of antibodies to testosterone-3-BSA, estrone-17-BSA, cortisol-21-BSA, and aldosterone-

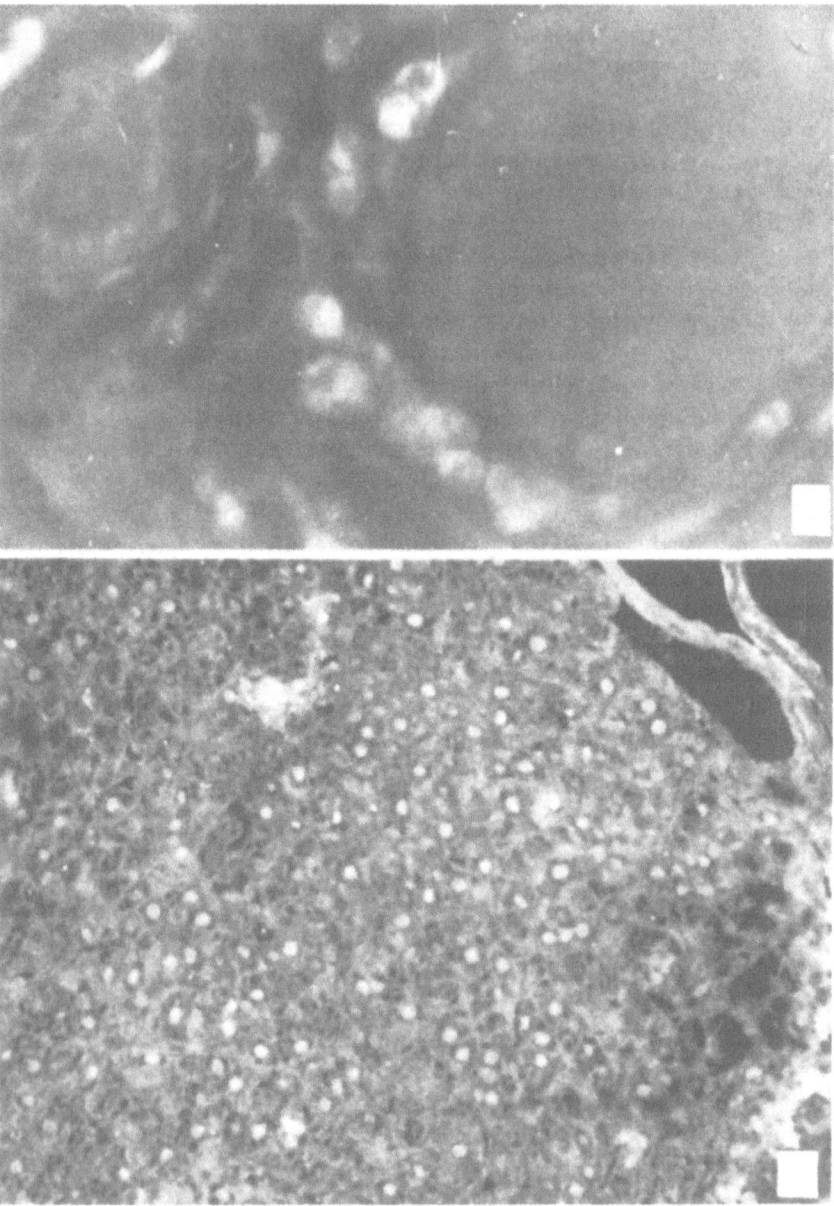

Fig. 10. Top: Section of mature rat ovary stained with fluorescein-labeled anti-C-2-EHSA globulin. Perifollicular cells showed green fluorescence of the cyptoplasm. Bottom: Section of ovary FSH-stimulated mature rat stained with fluorescein-labeled anti-C-2-EHSA globulin. *From* Goodfriend et al. 1961. *Can. J. Biochem. Physiol.*, 39:970. Reproduced by permission of the National Research Council of Canada.

TABLE 3

Inhibition of Exogenous Estrone in Immature Rats

Uterine to body (U/B)[a] ratios obtained with:[b]

Group No.	Buffered saline	0.2 μg estrone	0.2 μg estrone +0.8 ml anti-serum to HSA	0.2 μg estrone +0.8 ml anti-serum to C-17-EHSA
1	0.83	1.38	1.27	0.89
2	0.72	0.82	1.24	1.21
3	0.72	0.96	1.27	0.92
4	0.84	0.98	1.23	0.91
5	0.80	1.29	1.13	0.82
6	0.86	0.81	0.88	0.92
7	0.75	0.96	0.93	0.70
8	0.77	1.31	1.06	0.76
9	0.71	1.10	0.96	0.68
10	0.77	0.94	1.04	0.87
11	0.73	1.16	0.93	0.71
12	0.78	1.14	1.29	0.69
13	0.79	1.14	0.93	0.87
14	0.70	0.93	1.07	0.80
15	0.72	1.00	0.98	0.68
16	–	–	1.04	0.80
17	–	–	0.98	1.06
18	–	–	1.19	0.96
19	–	–	0.94	1.04
20	–	–	0.95	0.72
21	–	–	1.02	0.68
22	–	–	–	0.91
23	–	–	–	0.97
24	–	–	–	0.85
Average U/B	0.76	1.06	1.05	0.85
Standard deviation[c]	±0.051	±0.174	±0.126	±0.122

[a]U represents the uterine weight in milligrams; B represents the body weight in grams.
[b]All solutions were made up in buffered saline and administered intraperitoneally in 2-ml volumes.
[c]The "pooled" standard deviation for the U/B values listed in the last two columns is ±0.124, which leads to a value of $P < 0.001$ in terms of student's t statistics (t = 5.4).
After Goodfriend and Sehon. 1961b. Can. J. Biochem. Physiol., 39:963. Reproduced by permission of the National Research Council of Canada.

21-BSA to appropriate test animals neutralized the biologic effects ordinarily caused by exogenous administration of the corresponding steroid hormones. An example of their findings is shown in Table 4. In immature mice, passive transfer of antiserum to estrone by intraperitoneal injection along with subcutaneous injection of estrone over a period of 3 days resulted in a complete depression to normal levels of uterine to

TABLE 4

Effect of Estrone and of Estrone + Antiserum to E-17-BSA on the Ratio of Uterine Weights to Final Body Weights of Immature Mice

Total dose of estrone (μg)		Total volume of antiserum to E-17-BSA (ml)	Uterine weight (mg)	Ratio of uterine weight to final body weight (mg/g)
—	+	—	9.7	0.80
0.30	+	—	34.3	3.20
0.30	+	0.6	8.6	0.81
—	+	0.6	6.9	0.59

Each group consisted of either 5 or 6 mice

Analysis of variance		
Source of variation	Degrees of freedom	Ratio of uterine weight to final body weight (mean square)
(1) Estrone Concentrations	1	10.2574
(2) Anti-E-17-BSA Concentrations	1	10.1011
(3) Interaction of (1) and (2)	1	7.1395[a]
(4) Residual	18	.0313

[a]Significant; $P < 0.01$.
After Neri et al. 1964. Endocrinology, 74:594.

body weight ratios. The inhibition of estrogenic activity was shown to be specific inasmuch as passive transfer of the same antiserum to estrone did not prevent the increases in seminal vesical and levator ani to body weight ratios by exogenous testosterone.

Neri et al. (1964) have stressed that the anti-hormonal activity of steroid-specific antiserum does not manifest itself immediately but becomes evident only in long-term assays. The difference in our findings and those of the Columbia group may be more apparent than real, since we mixed estrone and anti-estrone antiserum in vitro, which would favor the *rapid* formation of potentially biologically inactive estrone-antibody complexes. The formation of such inactive steroid-antibody complexes would be expected to proceed relatively slowly when the two reagents are injected separately in vivo. Regarding the question posed by Neri et al. (1964) concerning the importance of timing in the administration of the anti-steroid antiserum versus its dosage, we wonder if the important question here is the level of circulating anti-steroid antibodies. In this connection it would be of interest to determine if an early anti-hormonal activity to exogenously administered steroid would be observed in animals actively hyperimmunized with steroid-protein conjugates.

Immunoassay of Steroid Hormones

The steroid-specific antibodies were shown to represent a heterogeneous population of 'molecules, heterogeneous in the sense that they were able to accommodate, in varying degree, a spectrum of heterologous steroids. Such heterogeneity would of course present no practical difficulty in connection with the assay of steroid solutions in which the identity of the steroid was known, but might do so in the case of solutions containing qualitatively unidentified steroid (s). To obviate this difficulty, Lieberman et al. (1959) have suggested the preparation of monospecific antibodies by immunoabsorption of antisera directed to a given steroid, with conjugates prepared with heterologous steroids.

Pressman (1957) has demonstrated that the anti-hapten antibody site may be complementarily adapted to different orientations of the hapten with respect to the carrier protein moiety of the immunizing conjugate. One might expect similar differences in the orientation of a given steroid hapten coupled to macromolecules such as proteins because of heterogeneity in the micro environments of the steroid residues within different regions of the protein carriers. The use of steroid-protein conjugates as antigens might therefore be expected to result in the production of anti-steroid antibody preparations, with a high degree of configurational heterogeneity of their combining sites. This would allow for cross-reactions with heterologous steroids due to their possession of structural features closely related to those of the steroid in the conjugates used for immunization.

We recognize that this approach may overemphasize the importance of orientation in determining the heterogeneity in the antibody combining sites of the anti-steroid antibodies. It is possible that appreciable cross-reactivity of such antibodies is inevitable irrespective of the orientation of the steroid with respect to the carrier owing to the possibility, suggested by Klopstock et al. (1964), that the immunodominant locus of all steroid molecules may reside in the lyophobic region of cyclopentanoperhydrophenanthrene, with the peripheral substituents exerting only secondary influence. However, some orientations may favor the immune response specific to such peripheral substituents, and it would be of interest in this connection to compare the heterogeneity of antibodies produced to a given steroid when attached to a protein on the one hand, and a chemically more homogeneous macromolecule, such as a synthetic polypeptide, on the other.

With regard to techniques for immunoassay of steroids, as such, some of the methods employed by us and by the Columbia group in those preradioimmunoassay days, may deserve further consideration. We have in mind, in particular, hapten inhibition of the turbidimetric and passive hemagglutination reactions, because of their simplicity and rapidity.

Figure 11 shows the standard curve obtained for 17α-ethynylestradiol-17β by hapten-inhibition of the turbidimetric reaction and the results of an assay of a solution of 4 μg of the steroid/ml (Goodfriend and Sehon, 1961a). It is clear from the curve that concentrations of the estrogens between 0.1 and 1 μg/ml could also be assayed by this method, and still greater sensitivity might be attained by further refinements in technique.

Beiser and Erlanger (1967) demonstrated a higher order of sensitivity for their method of steroid-hapten inhibition of the hemagglutination reaction. As little as 0.05 μg/ml of testosterone and estradiol-17β could be detected.

In spite of the virtues of the aforementioned techniques and of other classical methods of assay which might be mentioned, it seems to us that the future of immunoassay of steroids lies with the more recently developed, highly sensitive, and quantitative immunologic techniques, such as the radioimmunoassay methods, which will be reported upon at this symposium.

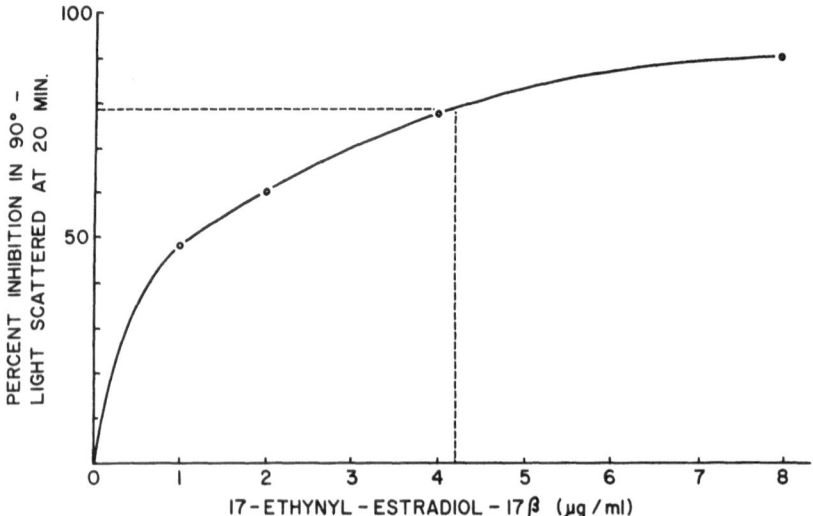

Fig. 11. Plot of percentage inhibition of turbidity due to C-17-EBSA-anti-C-17-EHSA reaction obtained for various concentrations of 17α-ethynyl estradiol-17β. The broken horizontal line represents the percentage inhibition obtained with a solution of ethynyl estradiol of concentration about 4.0 μg/ml. *From* Goodfriend and Sehon. 1961. *Can. J. Biochem. Physiol.*, 39:957. Reproduced by permission of the National Research Council of Canada.

MECHANISM OF FORMATION OF ANTIBODIES TO STEROIDS AND OTHER LOW-MOLECULAR-WEIGHT METABOLITES

As noted earlier, at the time of these studies only two instances had been reported of the experimental production of antibodies to low-molecular-weight metabolites normally present in the host. The induction of steroid-specific antibodies provided yet another demonstration of this phenomenon. A central question posed by these findings concerns the mechanism governing the formation of such antibodies in the face of the accepted maxim that antibodies are not normally produced against the host's own constituents, and, in particular, against common, low-molecular-weight metabolites. Obviously, this question is intimately related to the as yet unsolved and intriguing problems of the underlying mechanism determining the immunogenicity of a macromolecule, the breakdown of naturally acquired immunologic tolerance of autologous macromolecules, and the genetic factors controlling immunologic responsiveness and specificity.

Before attempting any speculations, it would seem appropriate to outline some of the current immunologic views relevant to these problems. In line with the suggestion of Sela (1969), it is necessary to distinguish the following attributes of an antigen:

(1) The immunogenicity of a substance, which represents its capacity to provoke an immune response: the immunogen is then the immunologically active moiety produced by the "processing" of the antigen, probably by phagocytic cells, and might be an antigenic fragment or one of these fragments hooked onto an RNA molecule of the processing cell (Gottlieb, 1968, 1969; Green et al., 1968; Humphrey, 1969).

(2) The antigenic specificity of a given group or groups of a molecule responsible for the "specific" interaction of the molecule with antibodies possessing an appropriate, configurationally complementary combining site. As pointed out in Dr. Pressman's lecture at this symposium, antibody preparations are in general highly heterogeneous with respect to their binding affinity. This property reflects configurational differences of the combining sites of the different antibody molecules within a given preparation, and is the basis for the interaction of cross-reacting systems, thus limiting the discriminating power, i.e., the "specificity" of immunologic techniques used for the qualitative and/or quantitative determination of antigens or haptens.

(3) The essential participation of the "carrier" molecule in the induction of the synthesis of antibodies with anti-hapten specificity. This has been amply documented since the pioneering studies of Landsteiner (Landsteiner, 1945; Green et al., 1968; Levine et al., 1968), and there is

increasing evidence favoring the view that antibody formation must include recognition for the carrier as well as for the hapten, and that such recognition events may involve two interacting cells or two separate events on the same cell (Landy and Braun, 1969). In all likelihood, the haptenic residue.acquires the ability to trigger off immunocytes with configurationally complementary "receptor groups" into active antibody synthesis by its prior incorporation into an immunogenic moiety, in which it plays the role of the immunodominant locus (Landy and Braun, 1969).

According to Mitchison (see Boak et al., 1969) and others (Dresser, 1962; Frei et al., 1965), a good case can be made for the hypothesis that direct exposure of lymphocytes to antigen leads to tolerance, whereas exposure to the immunogen via the macrophage leads to immunity. Thus, the lymphocyte would not be activated into antibody synthesis by low-molecular-weight soluble compounds and must be considered tolerant to these compounds. The termination of this tolerance by immunization with hapten-carrier conjugates could then be visualized as follows: The hapten-carrier conjugate is an artificial device to incorporate the haptenic residue as the immunodominant moiety into an immunogen, which contains determinants cross-reacting with natural antibodies or which are capable of inducing synthesis of antibodies with secondary specificities not directly related to the hapten. These secondary antibodies could then combine with the hapten-carrier conjugates and thus increase the local concentration of the antigen through formation of complexes. The latter would in turn be processed by macrophages into immunogenic materials possessing sufficient binding capacity for the anti-hapten receptor groups on appropriate lymphocytes, and thus stimulate the latter into active synthesis of antibodies with anti-hapten specificities.

This hypothetical framework seems to provide a general and plausible explanation for the observations reported at this symposium and in the recent immunologic literature, that antibodies can be elicited against normal metabolites, such as steroids, 5-hydroxyindole-3-acetic acid, serotonin (Ranadive and Sehon, 1967a,b), nucleotides (Plescia and Braun, 1968; Sela, 1969), and even glucose (Rude et al., 1966), on condition that these molecules are presented to the immunologic machinery in the form of hapten-carrier conjugates.

REFERENCES

Astwood, E. B. 1938. A six-hour assay for the quantitative determination of estrogen. Endocrinology, 23:25–31.

Beiser, S. M., B. F. Erlanger, F. J. Agate, and S. Lieberman, 1959. Antigenicity of steroid-protein conjugates. Science, 129:564–565.

———— and B. F. Erlanger. 1967. Estimation of steroid hormones by an immunochemical technique. Nature (London), 214:1044–1045.

Boak, J. L., E. Kolsch, and N. A. Mitchison. 1969. Immunological tolerance and inhibition by hapten. *In* Landy, M., and W. Braun, eds., Immunological Tolerance, 98–109, New York, Academic Press, Inc.

Clutton, R. F., C. R. Harington, and M. E. Yuill. 1938. Studies in synthetic immunochemistry. III. Preparation and antigenic properties of thyroxyl derivatives of proteins, and physiological effects of their antisera. Biochem. J., 32:1119.

Dresser, D. W. 1962. Specific inhibition of antibody production. II. Paralysis induced in mice by small quantities of protein antigen. Immunology, 5:378–388.

Erlanger, B. F., F. Borek, S. M. Beiser, and S. Lieberman. 1957. Steroidprotein conjugates. I. Preparation and characterization of conjugates of bovine serum albumin with testosterone and cortisone. J. Biol. Chem., 228:713–727.

———— F. Borek, S. M. Beiser, and S. Lieberman. 1959. Steroid-protein conjugates. II. Preparation and characterization of conjugates of bovine serum albumin with progesterone, deoxycorticosterone, and estrone. J. Biol. Chem., 234:1090–1094.

Faleck, B. 1959. Site of production of oestrogen in rat ovary as studied in micro-transplants. Acta Physiol. Scand., 47: Suppl. 163.

Frei, P. C., B. Benacerraf, and G. J. Thorbeke. 1965. Phagocytosis of the antigen, a crucial step in the induction of the primary response. Proc. Nat. Acad. Sci. USA, 53:20–23.

Goodfriend, L. 1960. Antigenicity of estrone-protein conjugates. Ph.D. Thesis. McGill University, Montreal, Canada.

———— and A. H. Sehon. 1958. Preparation of the estrone-protein conjugate. Can. J. Biochem. Physiol., 36:1177–1184.

———— and A. H. Sehon. 1960. Antigenicity of estrone-protein conjugates. Nature (London), 185:764–766.

———— and A. H. Sehon. 1961a. Antibodies to estrone-protein conjugates. I. Immunochemical studies. Can. J. Biochem. Physiol., 39:941–960.

———— and A. H. Sehon. 1961b. Antibodies to estrone-protein conjugates. II. Endocrinological studies. Can. J. Biochem. Physiol., 39:961–965.

———— A. Leznoff, and A. H. Sehon. 1961. Antibodies to estrone-protein conjugates. III. Tissue localization of estrogens. Can. J. Biochem. Physiol., 39:967–971.

Gottlieb, A. A. 1968. The antigen-RNA complex. *In* Plescia, O. J., and W. Braun, eds. Nucleic Acids in Immunology, 471–486, New York, Springer Verlag.

———— 1969. Macrophage nucleoprotein; nature of the antigenic fragment. Science, 165:592–594.

Green, I., B. B. Levine, W. E. Paul, and B. Benacerraf. 1968. The relationship of the hapten to the carrier in the induction and specificity of the immune response. *In* Plescia, O. J., and W. Braun, eds., Nucleic Acids in Immunology, 288–300, New York, Springer Verlag.

DISCUSSION

B. CALDWELL.   What role does the carrier play in the formation of specific antibodies to haptens? I am thinking in particular about the use of inert carriers such as charcoal, which reportedly are able to act in the same manner as the various carrier proteins when steroids are adsorbed onto the surface.

L. GOODFRIEND.   Of course, I do not have the answer to that. Speaking speculatively, I would say that the immunologic apparatus has recognized charcoal as a "carrier" which winds up in macrophages, with steroid and perhaps some steroid-protein complexes adsorbed to the surface.

W. ROSNER.   I wonder if you would comment on using as antigens, steroids coupled to synthetic peptides. Polylysine is readily available and one could then couple as many or as few moles of steroid per mole of peptide as desired. Would you expect either qualitatively or quantitatively better antibodies using this arrangement?

L. GOODFRIEND.   Given the possibility of heterogeneity in antibody combining sites due to heterogeneity in orientation of hapten with respect to carrier, one might expect less antibody site heterogeneity using hapten coupled to a structurally less complex carrier. I wonder if comparative studies of this kind have been done . . . perhaps Dr. Pressman can throw some light on this?

D. PRESSMAN.   The question then is, "Does a simplified carrier give a simplified antibody response?" Several studies have been carried out on this subject and without going into great detail, I will say that using simplified repeating unit carriers does not seem to give you better results in getting homogeneous antibodies than the complex antigens that have been more commonly used, such as BSA or KLH (bovine serum albumin, keyhole limpet hemocyanin).

J. KOWAL.   I wonder if you would care to speculate in your antibody studies in vitro, whether you think the antibodies were able to penetrate the membrane of the mitochondria to localize the steroids within the mitochondria.

L. GOODFRIEND.   They might be able to penetrate.

J. KOWAL.   I was speaking primarily in terms of its usefulness in localizing steroids within a cell at various stages of biosynthesis.

Humphrey, J. H. 1969. The fate of antigen and its relationship to the immune response. *In* Sorkin, E., ed. Antibiot. Chemother., 15:7–23.

Klopstock, A., M. Pinto, and A. Rimon. 1964. Antibodies reacting with steroid haptens. J. Immun., 92:515–519.

Landsteiner, K. 1945. The Specificity of Serological Reactions. Cambridge, Mass., Harvard University Press.

Landy, M., and W. Braun, eds. 1969. Immunological Tolerance. New York, Academic Press, Inc.

Levine, B. B., I. Green, and B. Benacerraf. 1968. The genetic control of the immune response to hapten-poly-L-lysine conjugates in guinea pigs. *In* Plescia, J. O., and W. Braun, eds., Nucleic Acids in Immunology, 277–287, New York, Springer Verlag.

Lieberman, S., B. F. Erlanger, S. M. Beiser, and F. J. Agate. 1959. Steroid-protein conjugates: Their chemical, immunochemical and endocrinological properties. Recent Progr. Hormone Res., 15:165–196.

Mooser, H., and R. K. Grilichess. 1941. Immunisierungsversuche mit steroiden. Schweitz. Z. allgem. Pathol. u. Bakteriol., 4:375–380.

Neri, R. O., S. Tolksdorf, S. M. Beiser, B. F. Erlanger, F. J. Agate, and S. Lieberman. 1964. Further studies on the biological effects of passive immunization with antibodies to steroid-protein conjugates. Endocrinology, 74:593–598.

Plescia, O. J., and W. Braun, eds. 1968. Nucleic Acids in Immunology, New York, Springer Verlag.

Pressman, D. 1957. Molecular complementariness in antigen-antibody systems. *In* Pauling, L., and H. A. Itano, eds., Molecular Structure and Biological Specificity, 1, Washington, D.C., Publication No. 2, American Institute of Biological Sciences.

Ranadive, N. S., and A. H. Sehon. 1967a. Antigenicity of 5-hydroxyindole-3-acetic acid, a derivative of serotonin. Canad. J. Biochem., 45:1681–1699.

———— and A. H. Sehon. 1967b. Antibodies to serotonin. Canad. J. Biochem., 45:1701–1710.

Rude, E., O. Westphal, E. Hurwitz, S. Fuchs, and M. Sela. 1966. Synthesis and antigenic properties of sugar-polypeptide conjugates. Immunochemistry, 3:137–151.

Sela, M. 1969. Antigens and antigenicity. Naturwissenschaften, 56:206–211.

Sheldon, J. M., N. Fell, J. H. Johnston, and H. A. Howes. 1941. A clinical study of histamine azoprotein in allergic disease: A preliminary report. J. Allerg., 13:18–30.

Vallery-Radot, P. 1957. Allergic manifestations of the female patient from puberty to menopause. J. Mount Sinai Hosp., N. Y., 24:444–455.

Westphal, U., and B. D. Ashley. 1958. Steroid protein interactions. IV. Influence of functional groups in Δ^4-3-ketosteroids on interaction with serum albumin and β-lactoglobulin. J. Biol. Chem., 233:57–62.

L. GOODFRIEND.   It is an interesting idea which might work using ferri-tin-labeled antibodies. However, it would probably be more realistic, at the present stage, to apply a technique such as complement-fixation immunoassay (Hamburger, R. N. 1966. Chloramphenicol-specific anti-body. *Science*, 152:203) for subcellular localization of steroids, in view of the minute amounts of steroid which would be involved.

J. KOWAL.   In the studies in vivo, was the inhibition seen only when the antibody and the antigen were mixed together? To determine whether the estrogen effect was blocked by the antibody, did you inject these into two separate sites?

L. GOODFRIEND.   I did not try it. Apparently, you would not get an early neutralization, as Neri et al. (1964)* have shown. I do not think that you *can* get an early response under their conditions because *time* is required for antibodies to get into the circulation and interact with the administered steroid to form complexes. In our own studies, we formed the antibody-steroid complexes in vitro, reducing the latent period for formation of inactive complexes essentially to zero.

R. NERI.   Our observations suggested that anti-hormonal effects result-ing from the administration of steroid-specific antibodies do not manifest themselves immediately. In the tests involving daily treatment for several days (estrogen and androgen assays), hormone inhibition by specific antibodies occurred. However, in the acute eosinophil and electrolyte assays in which we attempted to demonstrate anti-hormonal properties of antisera to estrone-17-BSA and aldosterone-21-BSA respectively, no inhi-bition was detected. When the animals were pretreated with the appropriate antisera for 3 days prior to the day of the test, inhibition was found.

L. GOODFRIEND.   I would expect in view of your results and our own that you would see an early inhibition effect in animals directly hyper-immunized with steroid-protein conjugate, since they might contain sufficiently high levels of anti-steroid antibodies *already in their circula-tion.*

A. R. MIDGLEY.   With regard to your localization of estradiol in cellular sites, could you give us some additional information on the levels of autofluorescence and on the techniques used for fixation?

L. GOODFRIEND.   We certainly cannot say from our data that we have localized cellular sites of formation of estrone or the estrogens since, as we have emphasized, some central aspects of this study were incomplete:

* Neri et al. 1964. Further studies on the biological effects of passive immunization with antibodies to steroid-protein conjugates. Endocrinology, 74: 593–598.

using anti-estrone antiserum, we localized *some* component in cells which one would expect to be the site of estrogen biosynthesis, but this, of course, might be coincidental with other processes. As to technique, we used *unfixed, frozen* sections to avoid, or at least to minimize, precisely this problem of diffusion. We also observed autofluorescence but could distinguish this from fluorescence due to the tagged antiserum. As to controls: none of the ovaries from immature rats showed specific fluorescence. While two untreated rats were negative when stained with fluorescein tagged anti-bovine γ-globulin, only one untreated mature rat gave positive fluorescence, although the tissues from both animals were treated identically. In contrast, all of the FSH-stimulated rat ovaries were positive.

S. GROSS. Haferkamp and co-workers (1968) * described localization of fluorescein-labeled T-3 antibodies. Stumpf has demonstrated localization in lyophilized material by radioautography. We have seen estradiol antibody labeled with ^{125}I in trophoblasts. One should not fix the sections. It is unlikely that washing briefly will remove all detectable hydrophobic steroid from cell constituents after coupling with antibody. Fixatives are undesirable for localization of biologically active materials in cells. Such harsh treatment is merely useful for morphologic identification. Autoradiographic preparations need not even be stained. Details are discernible by phase-contrast observation.

---

* Haferkamp et al. 1968. Experimental and immunological investigations of biologic effects produced by hormones. Int. Arch. Allergy, 33:528–534.

3

SPECIFICITIES OF STEROID ANTIBODIES

Stanley J. Gross

Department of Pathology
University of California, Irvine
California College of Medicine
Irvine, California

INTRODUCTION

Numerous disciplines borrow concepts and methods from the field of immunology. None has found wider application than the principles which underlie immune assay of important protein molecules in body fluids. Certain nonprotein substances, e.g., α-DNP- (lys)$_7$, arsanilic acid azo-D are able, despite low molecular weight and initial absence of reactive groups, to induce antibody formation (Kabat, 1968). Steroids are not immunogenic by themselves but can serve effectively as haptens. Lieberman, Goodfriend, and their colleagues made the significant original observations without which we would have very little to discuss at this symposium (Beiser et al., 1959; Erlanger et al., 1957, 1959; Goodfriend and Sehon, 1958, 1961a and 1961b; Lieberman et al., 1959).

It was shown that steroid-protein conjugates synthesized by Schotten-Baumann substitution or the mixed anhydride reaction (Erlanger et al., 1958; Goodfriend and Sehon, 1961a and 1961b) which attack important functional groups of the steroids are capable of raising antibodies. These distinguish the aromatic from the alicyclic A ring. However, cross reactivity within the major steroid classes is common, the immunologic specificities being less dependent on the individual steroid than on the particular carbonyl or phenol group occupied.

Since number and steric orientation of hydroxyl groups have been shown to be highly specific with respect to functional behavior of an estrogen at cellular targets, we hoped to render estrogens antigenic in a manner which would preserve the integrity of their polar groups. The phenolic hydroxyl function on C-3 enables the A ring to be coupled with diazobenzoic acid to yield estrogen azobenzoyl derivatives. The latter can be coupled to proteins through the azobenzoyl carboxyl by carbodiimide condensation retaining specificities of both C-3 and C-17 reactive groups (Gross et al., 1968) (Fig. 1). The large molecule, keyhole limpet hemo-

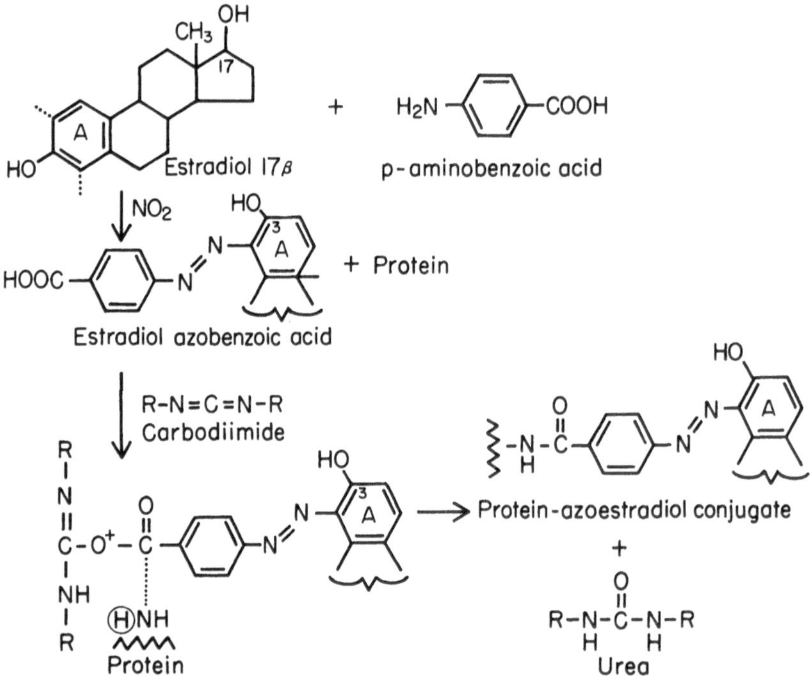

Fig. 1.   Synthesis of steroid azobenzoyl derivatives.

cyanin (KLH), serves as a suitable estradiol carrier for immunization. Antisera are tested against estradiol, estriol, and estrone coupled to human IgG.

MATERIALS AND METHODS

Synthesis of Steroid-Protein Conjugates

p-Aminobenzoic acid (PABA) is rapidly diazotized in the presence of an estrogen whose reactive phenolic C-3 function permits entry into the A ring at position 2 or 4 by the distal nitrogen atom. The resulting azosteroid is coupled to a protein through the azobenzoyl carboxyl by condensation with a soluble carbodiimide.*

PABA (137 mg) is dissolved in 1.0 N HCl (10 ml). The beaker is cooled with crushed ice for 5 minutes and 20 percent $NaNO_2$ (100 mg) is added while stirring. The temperature is not permitted to rise above 5°C. When all nitrite has been added (slight excess) a pale blue spot develops rapidly on testing with wetted starch-iodide paper. Excess $NaNO_2$ is removed by sulfamic acid. The solution should become clear yellow. Diazotization requires 15 minutes, the pH never exceeding 1.0.

Crystalline estradiol, estriol, or estrone (100 mg) is dissolved in 90 percent methanol (25 ml). Diazotized PABA is added dropwise, the pH being maintained at 10 to 11. The final mixture is acidified with 0.1 N HCl to remove excess (soluble) PABA and side-reaction products. The azosteroid precipitate is recovered, triturated, and redissolved in 0.1 N NaOH. Centrifugation removes insoluble unreacted steroid. After repeating the acid and base cycle once, the azosteroid is extracted into a mixture of benzene and methanol (4:1) which is evaporated to dryness.

Crystalline azosteroid (25 mg) is added to a 1 percent saline solution containing 0.1 M carbodiimide (100 mg) and KLH or IgG (250 mg). The mixture is stirred until azosteroid has coupled and is dialyzed for 2 to 3 days at 3°C in 0.5 M sodium carbonate, pH 8.2, until color no longer appears in the dialysis solution. A final dialysis is performed against 0.9 percent NaCl for 24 hours. The preceding steps remove unreacted steroid and derivative molecules. Insoluble protein is removed by centrifugation. Protein determination is made on the colored supernatant containing steroid-protein conjugate. The concentration is adjusted to approximately 1 percent by spectral measurement at 280 mμ.

Analysis of Azobenzoyl Derivatives

Samples were initially examined by thin layer chromatography (TLC). Glass slides coated with silica G were spotted and developed with chloroform:ethyl acetate:acetic acid (40:60:50). Then slides were heated 10 minutes at 110°C, sprayed with concentrated H_2SO_4, and observed under ultraviolet light while charring. For quantitative spectral analyses, samples were further purified by preparative TLC on 10 by 14 cm glass plates coated with silica G. Development in one direction was done with ether:methanol:acetic acid (94:5:1). Material migrating as reference standard was scraped from the plate and recovered by original solvent (10 times volume). The structure as originally postulated has been confirmed by mass spectroscopy (Gross and Gray, in preparation).

---

* 1-cyclohexyl-3-(2-morpholinoethyl)-carbodiimide metho-*p*-toluenesulfonate.

Absorption spectra of derivatives and conjugates were measured on a Cary recording spectrophotometer using rectangular cells of 10 mm light path. Difference spectra were obtained with 0.2 cm cell paths. An Aminco-Bowman spectrophotofluorometer operated with a number 5 slit arrangement, yielding a spectral band pass of 22 mμ, was used for initial excitation and emission measurement (Gross and Gray, in preparation) and a 5233253 arrangement (band pass=11 mμ) for enhancement readings. A further diminution cut the signal without increase in resolution.

Immunization

Adult New Zealand rabbits were immunized with azoestradiol-KLH conjugates. Intravenous injections were done twice weekly for 2 weeks; the total dose was 30 mg. Blood was drawn by cardiac puncture 1 and 2 weeks after the last injection. Effective antisera have also been raised by a single subcutaneous injection of complete Freund's adjuvant containing 2.5 ml of 1 percent conjugate, blood being obtained 21 to 28 days later.

Antibody Purification

Aminoethylcellulose (500 mg) was coupled through its amino groups (Weliky et al., 1964) to azosteroid (100 mg) in the presence of N-N^1-dicyclohexylcarbodiimide as described for synthesis of steroid-protein conjugates. Antibodies were dissociated by 1 N HAc from the solid matrix used as a slurry.

Immunologic Analysis

Azosteroid-KLH antisera were tested against azosteroids coupled to human IgG. Quantitative precipitin tests were done in duplicate. Tubes containing increasing concentrations of antigen were incubated with 0.25 to 0.50 ml antiserum diluted 1:1 at 37°C for 1 hour and at 4°C for 60 hours. Precipitates were washed three times with cold saline, dissolved in 0.5 N NaOH and the total protein determined by the method of Lowry et al. (1951). Quantitative absorption experiments were done in the same manner. Increasing concentrations of steroid-IgG conjugates were used to absorb antisteroid-KLH sera and the latter were then tested with a standard concentration of homologous conjugate. For immunoelectrophoresis, glass slides were layered with 2 ml of 1.0 percent agar in 0.075 M veronal buffer, pH 8.6 (B2 buffer, Beckman Instruments). A total of 50 mA was delivered to six slides which were subsequently developed in a moist chamber for 12 to 72 hours at room temperature. Microimmunodiffusion experiments were done placing 1.5 cm square templates upon 0.5 ml agar (Gross and Tökes, 1968). Quenching of antibody fluorescence by azosteroid haptens was determined at an excitation wavelength of 280 mµ and emission determined at a wavelength of 350 mµ. Enhancement of hapten fluorescence by antibody was measured at wavelengths of 336 ·mµ for excitation and 380 mµ for emission.

RESULTS

Absorption Spectra

Initial spectra were obtained for crude azosteroids to determine the extent of substitution in proteins. Measurements were obtained before conjugation and after removal of azo derivatives from protein carriers by alkaline hydrolysis (Gross et al., 1968). The azosteroid derivatives have absorption maxima of 350 to 364 mµ in methanol and 344 mµ in bicarbonate or phosphate buffer, pH 8.6. The molar extinction coefficient of estradiol azobenzoic acid (AED) is 1,460 in methanol. Assuming that the value for AED chromophore is unchanged when coupled to protein, increased absorption by conjugate over that of untreated protein at 350 mµ is due to added steroid azobenzoyl groups. The absorbance at 350 mµ divided by the extinction coefficient yields the concentration of steroid residues. Subtraction of the latter from concentration of conjugate gives the molar concentration of protein constituent. Molar ratios calculated from spectral curves range from 4 to 30 and are similar to those derived from TLC.

Thin Layer Chromatography

The single qualitative difference between crude and purified azosteroids migrating on TLC is the presence of a substantial amount of material remaining at the origin of the former and none at the origin of the latter. In the chromatography of both, only one spot migrates. Its rate is almost as rapid as reference standard steroids (R_s=0.87) (Gross and Gray, in preparation). Relative mobilities of azoestradiol and azoestriol are identical to those of untreated estradiol and estriol standards. Bright yellow fluorescence of azosteroid after spraying with H_2SO_4 matched that of the standard steroid and remained entirely superimposed on the spot occupied by the migrating azo derivative seen under visible light. The colored material retained at the origin in TLC of crude samples did not fluoresce. Progesterone and testosterone treated with diazotized PABA migrated separately and in advance of the orange colored azo spot, suggesting that a major portion of these steroids did not react with diazo-PABA.

Treatment of steroid-proteins with 1.0 N NaOH at 100°C for two hours recovers hydrolytic azosteroids which migrate and fluoresce exactly as the original derivatives. Results were indicative of no major alteration in the steroid as a result of coupling. It follows that we can determine by TLC the minimum number of steroid residues per molecule of protein carrier (Table 1) (Gross et al., 1968).

TABLE 1
Molar Ratios of Representative Steroid-Protein Conjugates

	Protein	
Steroid	KLH	IgG
estradiol	29	19
estriol	25	20
estrone	27	5

Purification of Azoestradiol Antibodies

From 200 mg matrix 0 to 300 μg (5.0 ml serum) antibody is recovered by dilute acid (1 N HAc or 0.1 N HCl). The average recovery is 25 percent. The probable contribution of hydrophobic interactions at binding sites suggested the use of urea (4 to 8 M), pH 3.2 for dissociation. These experiments and studies measuring the reactivity of recovered proteins are in progress. Early data indicate specific binding to homologous steroid hapten and to diethylstilbestrol.

Quantitative Precipitation Reactions

Estradiol-IgG (20:1 molar ratio) precipitates 220 to 700 μg/ml antibody protein (Gross et al., 1968). In a recent experiment using an early anti-AED-KLH serum from the initial group of immunized rabbits, 354 μg/ml antibody was brought down by homologous hapten coupled to human IgG (Fig. 2). Antigen concentrations were determined spectrally. Although estrone was less highly coupled to carrier IgG than estradiol (Table 1), all dilutions of estrone conjugate failed to precipitate 50 percent as much antibody as estradiol-IgG. Estriol cross-reacts moderately in reactions with crude antibody. IgG standard, IgG treated with diazotized PABA, progesterone (or testosterone), and carbodiimide were negative. Quantitative absorption results with related conjugates further suggest the specificity of crude estradiol antisera for homologous hapten (Fig. 3). Quantitative hapten-inhibition studies were unsatisfactory probably because of restricted hapten solubility in neutral aqueous solution. For higher sensitivity and to calculate precise specificities of ster-

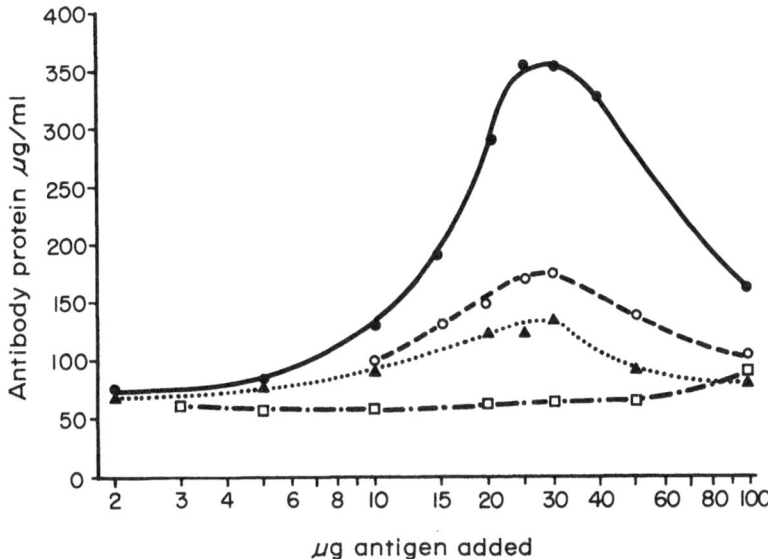

Fig. 2. Quantitative precipitin experiment in which a maximum of 354 μg/ml steroid antibody protein was precipitated from anti-steroid-KLH by azoestradiol-IgG (●——●). Azoestriol-IgG (○–––○); azoestrone-IgG (▲....▲); standard IgG (□·—·—·—□). Serum (0.25 ml) was diluted 1:1 and tested against increasing concentrations of IgG conjugates. Total volume was 1.25 ml. Supernatant was not examined.

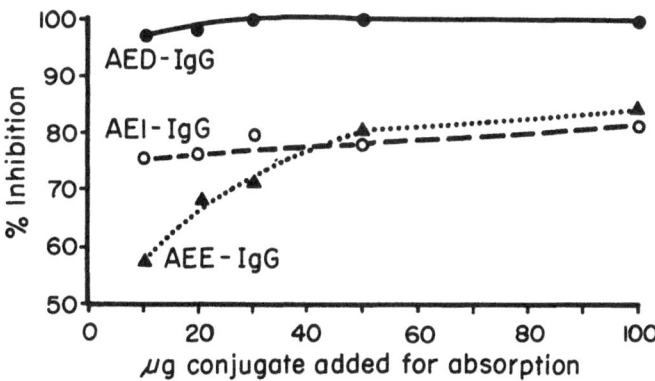

Fig. 3. Anti-estradiol-KLH was absorbed with increasing concentrations of different azosteroid-IgG in concentrations shown. Azoestradiol-IgG (●——●); azoestriol-IgG (○–––○); azoestrone-IgG ▲....▲).

oid-protein interactions, we sought a way which would not require drastic physical alteration of the steroid molecule or interfere with its binding kinetics.

Fluorescence Quenching Reactions

Perturbations of antibody (Haber and Richards, 1966; Velick et al., 1960) or hapten fluorescence (Dandliker and Levison, 1967; Yoo et al., 1967) consequent to their interaction can be very sensitive indicators of intensity and specificity of the interaction. A quantum of energy that would otherwise be emitted as fluorescence is absorbed by the smaller molecule instead of being directly dissipated into the solvent. The percent quenching of antibody fluorescence is proportional to the number of sites bound. Protein excited at a wavelength of 280 mμ emits maximally at a wavelength of 350 mμ $\pm$ 5 (tryptophan). This coincides with the absorption maximum of AED (Gross et al., 1968; Gross and Gray, in preparation) making possible energy transfer from the former to the latter. The efficiency of transfer from protein aromatic amino acid residues to the bound hapten can be calculated from comparisons of excitation and difference absorption spectra. In the absence of transfer, the excitation spectrum of hapten would coincide with the absorption spectrum of bound hapten. These studies with antibody and normal IgG are in progress.

Typical fluorescence quenching curves using crude antibody and AED are shown in Figure 4. Quenching maximum (Q max) was determined experimentally in hapten excess. The best values for Q max would yield an association constant (K_0) in agreement with one derived from equilibrium dialysis (for number of binding sites). However, constants determined by fluorescence quenching (assuming antibody valence of two) are useful when comparing related haptens in a given system. Since the antibody population can be assumed to be heterogeneous, the convenient sips equation (Karush, 1962) is used to describe the distribution or average K_0:

$$\log (r/n-r) = a \log c + a \log K_0$$

where r is the ratio of the number of moles of hapten bound per mole of antibody at c, the concentration of free hapten; n the maximum number of moles of hapten bound per mole of protein; and a the slope of the plot or index of heterogeneity. The value of testing impure azo or hydrazo (below) estradiol derivatives is 3.2×10^{-6}. Association constants are soon to be available for pure azo- and hydrazosteroids interacting with purified antibodies.

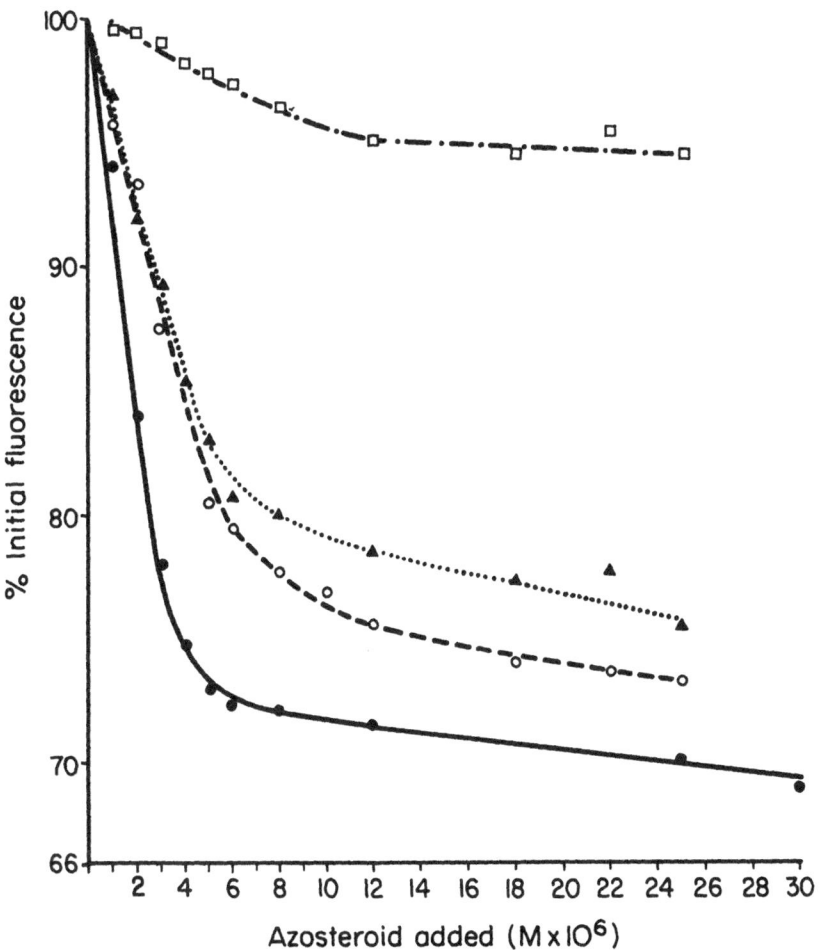

Fig. 4. Typical fluorescence quenching curves drawn as percent of maximum fluorescence observed after reacting azoestradiol-antibody IgG (1×10^{-8} *M*) with increasing concentrations of hapten. The fluorescence observed for solutions containing protein and azosteroid was subtracted from the value recorded for protein. Corrections were made for contributions of azosteroid, buffer, and dilution. Azoestradiol (●——●); azoestriol (○– – –○); azoestrone (▲ . . . . ▲). Contribution by nonspecific IgG binding of azosteroid is shown by azoestradiol + normal rabbit IgG (□ —·—·□). (Preimmune serum was no longer available).

Fluorescence Enhancement

For measurement of small quantities of hapten bound (either by dilution or lower association constants, e.g., with subunits of IgG) we have applied the technique of fluorescence enhancement (Stryer, 1965) using a highly fluorescent steroid which has some promise as a "reporter group" in the study of steroid-protein interactions. High natural fluorescence has been induced by reduction of azobenzoyl to hydrazobenzoyl derivatives. Synthesis and preliminary characterization have been described elsewhere (Gross and Gray, in preparation). Fluorescence excitation and emission maxima for hydrazoestradiol (HED) are 338 mμ and 388 mμ in 0.1 M phosphate buffer, pH 8.6. These small molecules when strongly bound to a protein in a nonpolar environment could be expected to acquire increased fluorescent energy (Stryer, 1965; and Sela and Mozes, 1966) if the donor (protein) and acceptor (HED) moieties meet the following spectroscopic criteria: (1) their absorption spectra

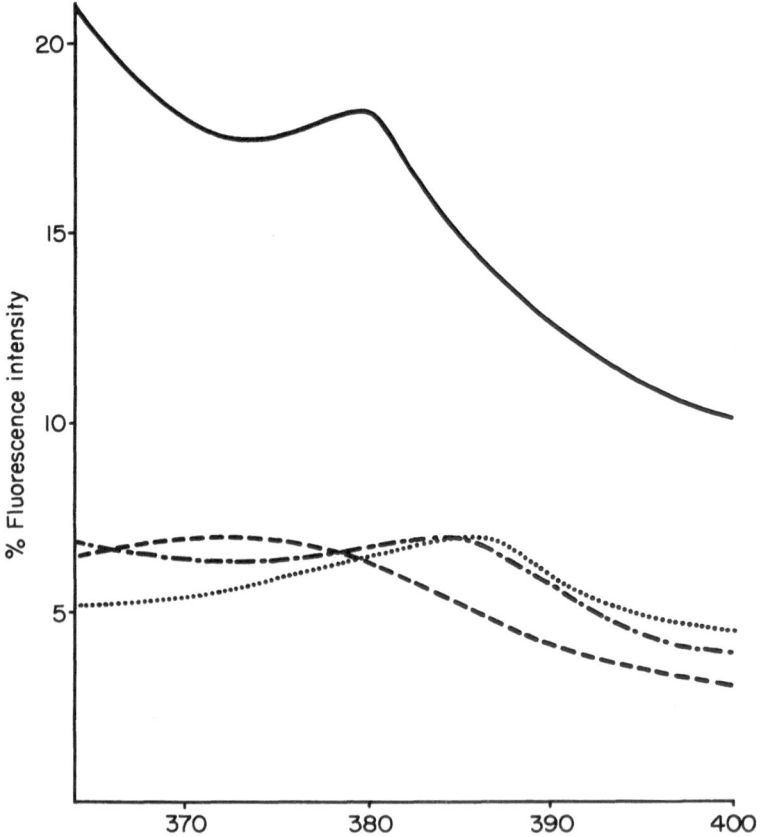

Fig. 5. Fluorescence emission spectra produced by excitation at a wavelength of 336 mμ. Note spectral shifts of HED interacting with antibody and normal IgG. HED + antibody (———); HED + normal IgG (—·—·—); HED (....); antibody IgG (– – –). Normal rabbit IgG curve coincided with that of antibody. Concentrations for HED (1 × 10⁻⁸ M) and proteins (5 × 10⁻⁸ M) were constant in each sample, corrections being made for dilution.

permit selective excitation of either chromophore, (2) the emission spectrum of the donor overlaps with absorption of the hydrazo acceptor chromophore, and (3) the acceptor is sufficiently fluorescent for detection of energy transfer.

Enhancement experiments have been done in hapten excess to protein excess using crude antibody IgG. Emission curves using an excitation wavelength of 336 mμ demonstrate a downward shift of emission

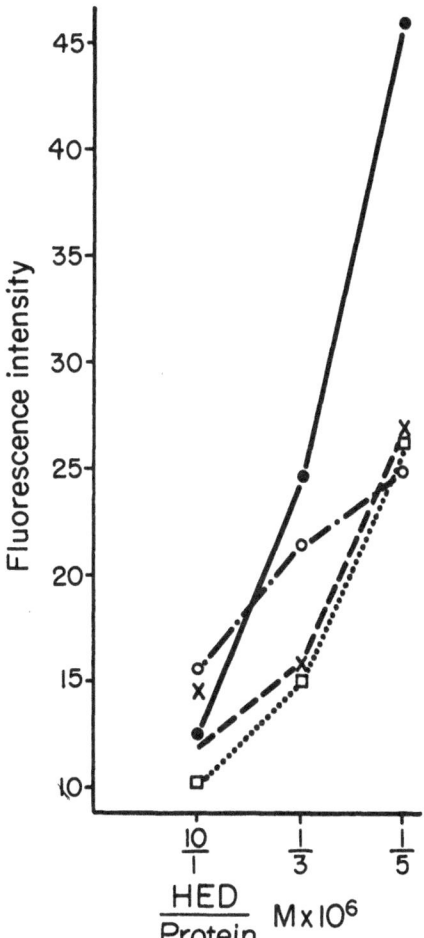

Fig. 6. Fluorescence enhancement of HED by azoestradiol antibodies at $\frac{\text{hapten}}{\text{protein}}$ concentrations ranging from $\frac{10 \times 10^{-6}}{1 \times 10^{-6}} M$ to $\frac{1 \times 10^{-6}}{5 \times 10^{-6}} M$. HED + antibody (●——●); HED + normal IgG (○ — · — · ○); antibody (x - - - x); normal IgG (□ . . . . □). Under conditions described in the text, HED coincides with buffer line above and parallel to abscissa.

(Fig. 5) . This experiment was done at a hapten concentration of 10^{-8} *M*. Similar changes were observed at 10^{-6} *M* (Fig. 6) . Quenching of antibody fluorescence by HED measured on the same samples (at the lower concentration) using an excitation wavelength of 284 mμ and reading intensity of emission at 350 mμ produced curves similar to those of AED. Quantitative experiments designed to compare purified estratriene derivatives are in progress.

The chemical changes produced with steroid derivative haptens have also been achieved with steroid-protein conjugates. Microgel immunodiffusion performed under nitrogen suggests immunologic identity as well as specificity of HED and AED determinants.

DISCUSSION

Earlier work demonstrated that it is readily possible for antibodies to distinguish between the aromatic and alicyclic A ring of steroids. However, the immunologic specificities of derivatives with blocked hydroxyl or carbonyl groups are seriously impaired. Thus testosterone coupled at C-17 cross-reacts more with a cortisone (C-21) derivative than with testosterone coupled at C-3 (Beiser et al., 1959) . Indeed, changing the hydroxyl at C-17 into a ketone considerably alters the immunologic specificity of the steroid hapten (Lieberman et al., 1959) .

It is not surprising that binding specificities of steroids within a major

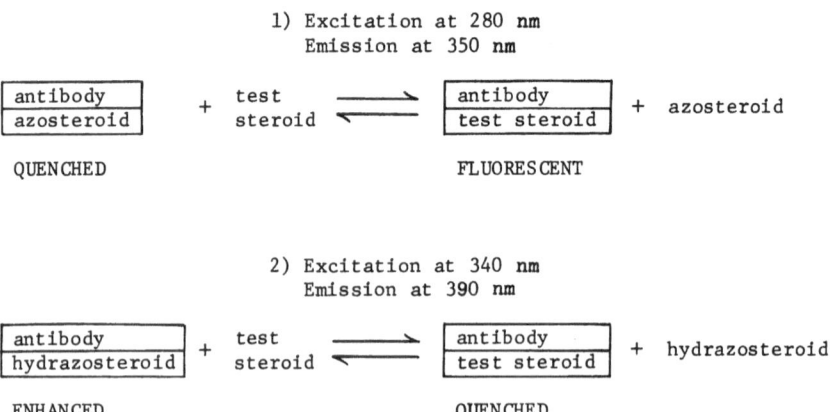

Fig. 7. Scheme for competition experiments in which quenching of fluorescence is accomplished by azosteroids (or hydrazoesteroids) whose absorption spectra overlap protein emission. The alternative approach utilizes fluorescence enhancement of hydrazosteroid by antibody.

class are related to the polar groups at C-3 and C-17 in a hydrophobic protein environment. Our experiments were designed to ascertain the specificity of estradiol antibodies for the homologous steroid. A reasonable specificity is demonstrated by crude antiserum. Improvement is expected with purified antibodies.

The potential usefulness of spectrophotofluorimetry as a very rapid and simple physicochemical means to assay standard estrogens by their competition with derivative molecules is shown in Figure 7. This scheme may also be used to probe the basic nature of hapten-protein binding. Since addition of a single hydroxyl at C-16 or conversion of the C-17 hydroxyl to the alpha stereoisomer are associated with the loss of biologic activity at cellular receptor proteins, estrogens constitute an ideal group of small, uncharged haptens to investigate the nature of strong interaction with large soluble receptor molecules.

REFERENCES

Beiser, S. M., B. F. Erlanger, F. J. Agate, and S. Lieberman. 1959. Antigenicity of steroid-protein conjugates. Science, 129:564–565.

Dandliker, W. B., and S. A. Levison. 1967. Investigation of antigen-antibody kinetics by fluorescence polarization. Immunochemistry, 5:171–183.

Erlanger, B. F., F. Borek, S. M. Beiser, and S. Lieberman. 1957. Steroid-protein conjugates. I. Preparation and characterization of conjugates of bovine serum albumin with testosterone and with cortisone. J. Biol. Chem., 228:713–727.

——— F. Borek, S. M. Beiser, and S. Lieberman. 1959. Steroid-protein conjugates. II. Preparation and characterization of conjugates of bovine serum albumin with progesterone, deoxycorticosterone and estrone. J. Biol. Chem., 234:1090–1094.

Goodfriend, L., and A. H. Sehon. 1958. Preparation of an estrone-protein conjugate. Canad. J. Biochem. and Physiol., 36:1177–1184.

——— and A. H. Sehon. 1961a. Antibodies to estrone-protein conjugates. I. Immunological studies. Canad. J. Biochem. Physiol., 39:941–960.

——— and A. H. Sehon. 1961b. Antibodies to estrone-protein conjugates. II. Endocrinological studies. Canad. J. Biochem. Physiol., 39:961–965.

Gross, S. J., and Z. Tökes. 1968. Red cell binding of gamma-heavy chains isolated from polyanylated anti-Rh$_0$ IgG. Nature (London), 219: 758–760.

——— D. H. Campbell, and H. H. Weetall. 1969. Production of antisera to steroids coupled to proteins directly through the phenolic A ring. Immunochemistry, 5:55–65.

Haber, E., and F. F. Richards. 1966. The specificity of antigenic recognition of antibody heavy chain. Proc. Roy. Soc. [Biol.], 166:176–187.

Kabat, E. A. 1968. Structural Concepts in Immunology and Immuno-chemistry. New York, Holt, Rinehart and Winston, Inc.

Karush, F. 1962. Immunologic specificity and molecular structure. *In* Taliaferro, W. H., and J. H. Humphrey, eds. Advances in Immunol-ogy, vol. 2,.1–40, New York, Academic Press, Inc.

Lieberman, S., B. F. Erlanger, S. M. Beiser, and F. J. Agate, Jr. 1959. Ster-oid-protein conjugates: Their chemical, immunochemical, and endo-crinological properties. Recent Progr. Hormone Res., 15:165–200.

Lowry, O. H., N. J. Rosebrough, A. L. Y. Farr, and R. J. Randall. 1951. Protein measurement with the Folin phenol reagent. J. Biol. Chem., 193:265–275.

Sela, M., and E. Mozes. 1966. The net electrical charge of antigens. Proc. Nat. Acad. Sci. USA, 55:445–452.

Stryer, L. 1965. The interaction of naphthalene dye with apomyoglobin and apohemoglobin. A fluorescent probe of non-polar binding sites. J. Molec. Biol., 13:482–495.

Velick, S. F., C. W. Parker, and H. N. Eisen. 1960. Excitation energy transfer and the quantitative study of the antibody hapten reaction. Proc. Nat. Acad. Sci. USA, 46:1470–1482.

Weliky, N., H. H. Weetall, R. V. Gilden, and D. H. Campbell. 1964. The synthesis and use of some insoluble immunologically specific adsor-bents. Immunochemistry, 1:219–229.

Yoo, T.-J., O. A. Roholt, and D. Pressman. 1967. Hapten binding activity in isolated light polypeptide chain from rabbit antibody. Cold Spring Harbor Symp. Quant. Biol., XXXII:117–118.

DISCUSSION

W. KELLY. I would like to make some comments on the specificity of some antibodies to steroids, and to report some work in progress in our laboratories. This work is being carried out in collaboration with the Columbia group and in particular with Dr. Zimmering. The Columbia group made antibodies to aldosterone and estriol in sheep several years ago. For aldosterone, the antigen was aldosterone-21-hemisuccinate conju-gated to bovine serum albumin. For the estriol, the antigen was the 16 (17) hemisuccinate conjugated to bovine serum albumin.

Figure 1 shows the competition between radioactive and nonradio-active aldosterone. We separate our bound from free steroid by precipita-tion with ammonium sulfate, centrifugation, and counting an aliquot of the supernatant fluid.

Figure 2 shows the same kind of curve for estriol.

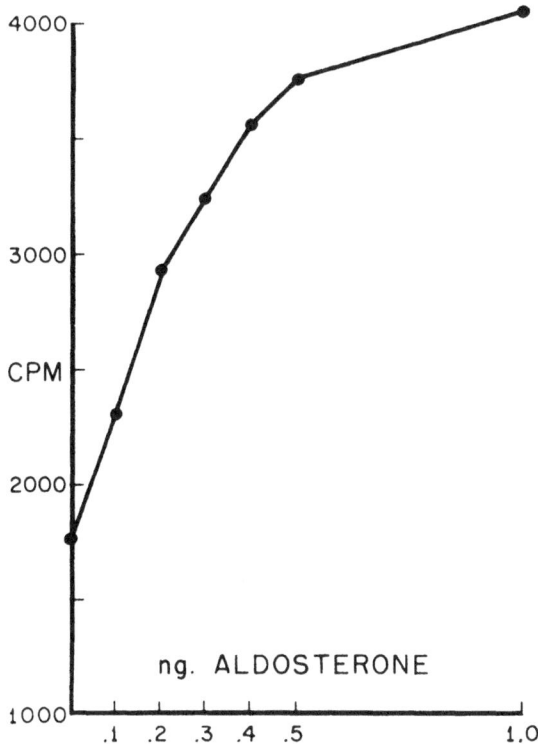

Fig. 1. Standard curve for aldosterone.

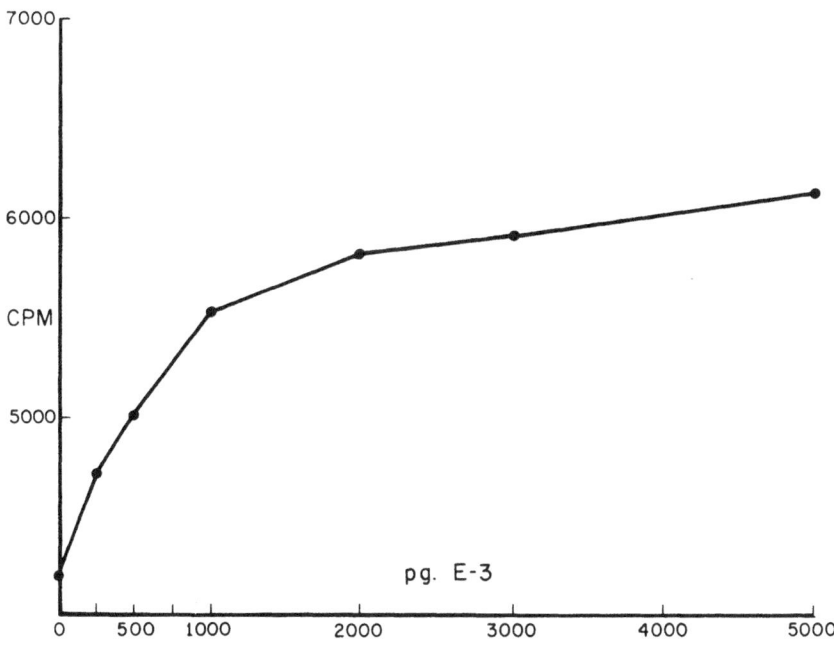

Fig. 2. Standard curve for estriol.

Table 1 gives the percentage of radioactive estriol displaced from the anti-estriol by various amounts of other steroids. The antibody to estriol is specific for estriol and cross-reacts with estrone and estradiol. The cross-reaction with Δ^4-3-ketosteroids and with the Δ^5-3β-hydroxy steroids is minimal.

Table 2 gives similar data for the anti-aldosterone. This antibody binds aldosterone and the γ-lactone derived at aldosterone equally. Cross-reaction with virtually any Δ^4-3-ketosteroid occurs. The steroids which do not have a 17α-hydroxyl group seem to cross-react more than those which do. The cross-reactivity with Δ^5-3β-hydroxy steroids is considerably less than with Δ^4-3-ketosteroids and the same is also true of the aromatic steroids. It would seem to us that these data indicate that the portion of the steroid which is most remote from the point of attachment to the antigen has a very important role in determining the specificity of the corresponding antibody.

J. KOWAL. I would appreciate it if Dr. Gross or someone else in the audience could summarize and speculate, for those of us who are neophytes in this field, about the specificity of these reactions.

S. GROSS. It would seem that there are probably two major aspects of specificity, at least with respect to estrogens. Free access to both the C-3 phenolic function and the C-17 reactive groups is highly important for

TABLE 1

Displacement of ^{3}H-Estriol from Anti-Estriol by Various Steroids

Steroid Added	cpm displaced/displaceable cpm $\times$ 100 (% cpm displaced)		
	1 ng	50 ng	500 ng
E-3	55	100	—
E-2	41	87	85
E-1	43	82	85
Progesterone	3	18	45
Testosterone	1	6	39
DOC	10	21	36
17-Hydroxyprogesterone	20	20	20
Androstenedione	4	1	23
Corticosterone	4	16	23
Cortisol	8	8	9
Dehydroisoandrosterone	11	15	35
Pregnenolone	16	—	38
17-Hydroxypregnenolone	3	6	5

TABLE 2

Displacement of ^{3}H-Aldosterone from Anti-Aldosterone by Various Steroids

Steroid Added	cpm displaced/displaceable cpm X 100 (% cpm displaced)		
	0.2 ng	1 ng	100 ng
Aldosterone	30	64	–
γ-lactone	32	56	94
Androstenedione	11	35	85
Progesterone	3	30	100
Corticosterone	3	20	100
Testosterone	6	16	90
DOC	4	13	94
17-Hydroxyprogesterone	4	7	73
Cortisol	8	15	49
Pregnenolone	5	4	28
Dehydroisoandrosterone	3	3	21
17-Hydroxypregnenolone	4	1	15
E-1	1	10	1
E-2	2	2	1
E-3	3	13	19

specificity. This pertains not only to binding with antibodies but also fixed biologic targets. The second important aspect of specificity clearly shown by Lieberman, Goodfriend, and their co-workers is the immune recognition of an aromatic versus an alicyclic A ring. Thus, one population of IgG recognizes the marked steric differences imparted by saturation of the A ring and at least one other population of IgG recognizes polar groups at both ends of the molecule. The relatively rigid steroid backbone and the portion linked to proteins are recognized by other molecules. However, it is obvious that the best assay will select the former population for study and avoid the use of BSA-absorption. If related haptens successfully inhibit, in a given concentration, a heterologous antibody, one is looking at the latter population of IgG. One last point: there are very few reactive sites on an uncluttered steroid molecule available for recognition and this factor can be used to advantage.

L. GOODFRIEND. I would concur with what Dr. Gross has just said. I think it is fully in line with the earlier data by the Columbia group and with our own. The available data indicate that among the steroids the estrogens, when functioning as haptens, produce the most specific antibodies, and this is what would be expected from general immunochemical experience.

In this connection, I would like to pose a question which relates to the specificity of the anti-estrogens. In the attempts to localize the estrogens in situ, you said, Dr. Midgley, that you had used anti-estrone or anti-estradiol antibodies. It is important to differentiate the estrone conjugates used. At what point did you conjugate the estrogens? From a standpoint of immunoassay this may not be terribly important, but from the standpoint of trying to localize in situ, we just do not know that the estrogens are attached to macromolecules, and at what position. In our own studies, and perhaps this is why we obtained some encouraging results, we assumed that a likely point would be via the phenolic ring. Accordingly, we used antisera prepared with the C-2 conjugate.

S. GROSS.   Those are very important points, and it would seem that in localization work one might prefer to use crude antisera instead of purified IgG which detects the polar groups. I must agree with Dr. Goodfriend. His view is entirely in accord with the data reported by those working with cellular target receptors which demonstrate very narrow binding specificity at the C-17 position.

E. GURPIDE.   We have obtained interesting results concerning the specificity of sheep antiserum against an antigen prepared by linking estriol ring D-hemisuccinate to bovine serum albumin. The antiserum was supplied to us by Dr. W. Kelly. As Figure 3 indicates, estriol-16-glucuronide (given to us by Dr. M. Levitz) and estradiol-17-glucuronide, as well as estrone and estradiol, displaced as much tritiated estriol from the bound to the free form as did equimolar amounts of estriol in the range of 0.5 to 6 ng. On the other hand, estrogens with a blocked phenolic hydroxyl group, such as estrone sulfate and the 3-methyl ethers of estrone, estradiol, and estriol, did not significantly change the binding of labeled estriol.

The reactivity of estriol-16-glucuronide with this antiserum was advantageously used to measure estrogens in urine without prior hydrolysis or extraction. Pregnancy urine samples diluted one thousand-fold and tested with this antiserum gave results that correlated very well with the estriol values obtained on the same urines after hydrolysis, extraction, and gas-liquid chromatography of the trimethylsilyl ethers. Urinary phenols did not cross-react or interfere in this assay; nonpregnancy urine samples at the same dilution used for testing pregnancy urine gave negligible blank values.

A. R. MIDGLEY.   I do not think that there is any necessary reason to believe that the steroid molecule once synthesized and stored within the cell needs to be fixed at any point. Although we did use for the estradiol localizations, antibodies which were generated against a C-17 derivative, our testosterone attempts were with antibodies against C-17 and C-3 derivatives, and neither one was successful.

A. SEHON.   I would like to take up again the question of the speed of these reactions. I think when we are talking about the speed of these reactions we must be definite also about the concentration of the reagents

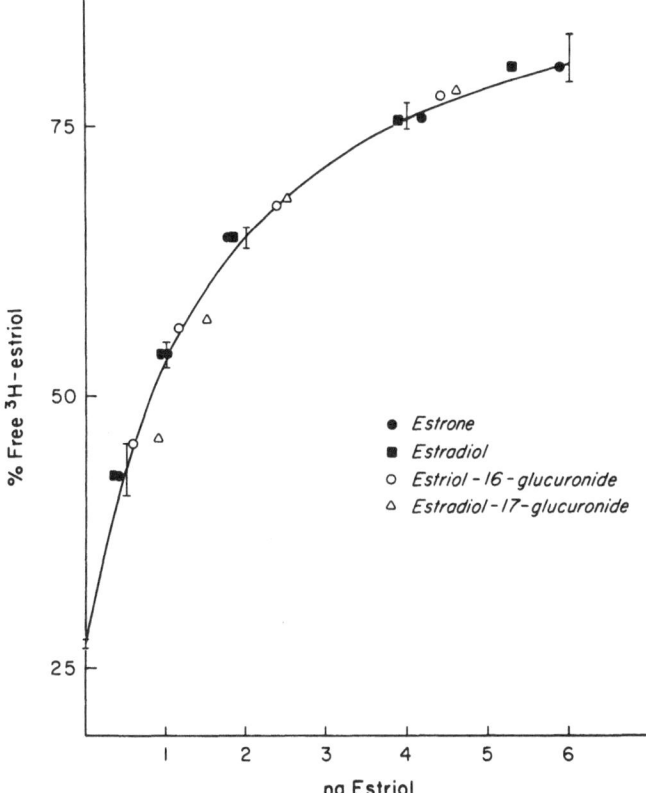

Fig. 3. Standard curves of various estrogens using an antiserum against estriol.

used. If you use concentrations of the order of 10^{-11} *M* your time of reaction of course would be a long one. We worked with 10^{-5} *M*, and of course there we talk about milliseconds. The half-life time of the reaction depends on the total concentration. Total for us is milliseconds. If you reduce your concentration by 10^6 then obviously it is milliseconds times 10^6, which is thousand seconds and so on.

S. GROSS. As I stated, the lowest concentrations we have used for enhancement reactions to date is 10^{-11} moles/ml or 10^{-8} *M*. Our experience has been entirely in accord with your comment that longer equilibration is necessary for dilute solutions. The fluorescence alterations we have described require only 10 minutes incubation and hence are ideal for simple assay. Overnight equilibration at 4°C in a screw cap vial may be more secure for low affinity IgG or diluted ligand.

J. FISHMAN. The specificity of the estrogen is due to the unique phenolic ring. Should not this specificity be challenged not with other steroids, but with nonsteroidal phenols which may be present in blood, such as catecholamines?

S. GROSS. That is correct.

J. KOWAL. In connection with my previous question, I was wondering if you could offer some conjecture about the future. Will preliminary separations of the various Δ^4-3-ketosteroids be necessary before measuring them this way? Could you picture a situation in which you will be able to develop specific antibodies?

S. GROSS. This is an interesting point. We personally have not assayed estrogen levels in serum or urine. Since crude antiserum can be used without risk of nonspecific interference just as effectively as lyophilized antibody IgG, perhaps one may extrapolate to an estrogen-competition experiment using concentrated, unextracted serum. This would be simple to ascertain.

B. CALDWELL. Perhaps the specificity of the antisera is not so important, because there certainly are methods available for absorbing free those antibodies directed against the steroid which you do not want to measure. Perhaps by processing the antisera with suitable methods, you can increase the specificity by getting rid of all the nonspecific antibodies.

S. GROSS. Investigators working with adsorbents might agree. For example, one could remove cross-reacting antibodies, retaining specific antibodies and inert IgG in the purified serum. However, for precise measurements and to probe steroid-protein binding one would require isolation of specific IgG.

G. NISWENDER. Most of our presentation tomorrow will involve the kind of things that Dr. Caldwell just alluded to. However, I think at this point it is probably germane to point out one thing. We are talking here about different types of cross-reactivity. In other words, if you actually have a heterogeneous antibody, that is one thing that possibly can be absorbed.

If, however, one is simply talking about differences in binding constants or differences in the affinity of various steroid hormones for the same population of antibodies, then of course absorption will never work. I think we will present some data, at least, with antiserum that we have produced, to show that the differences are due to differences in binding affinities between various steroid hormones, which do after all have the same basic structure, and it is not a problem of heterogeneous antisera.

S. GROSS. It is hazardous to talk about the average binding affinity of a mixed antibody population for a particular steroid hapten. Complexity is reduced by purifying the antiserum. All one sees in the techniques which have been discussed is the bound hapten. Differences are reflected in the K_0 values.

D. W. BULLOCK.   Dr. Arthur Malley and I, at the Oregon Regional Primate Research Center, were working on the conjugation of estradiol-17β to hemocyanin when Dr. Gross and his co-workers published their procedure (1968. *Immunochemistry*, 5:55–65) . It had occurred to us also, that coupling to the protein at a position on the steroid molecule remote from the biologically active sites would enhance the likelihood of obtaining specific antisera. We began with estradiol-17β recrystallized three times from methanol, acetone, and ethanol, and formed a conjugate with keyhole limpet hemocyanin by a method which differs only in some technical details from that of Gross et al. Antisera produced in rabbits had a titer of 0.48 mg antibody protein per ml and showed no cross-reaction with up to 30 μg of estrone in hapten-inhibition tests using the percutaneous anaphylaxis reaction of the guinea pig. Would it be possible to utilize this approach to conjungation for other steroids, for example, starting with 6β-OH-progesterone, and has Dr. Gross or anyone else tried this?

S. GROSS.   It may be possible to aromatize the A ring which would render it accessible for coupling or even enter the ring directly.

I. THORNEYCROFT.   If you did that, would you not lose your specificity?

S. GROSS.   One might salvage those antibodies directed to the functional groups.

I. THORNEYCROFT.   The higher specificity of our anti-estradiol antibodies seems to reside in the phenolic A ring, as other nonphenolic steroids do not tend to cross-react with them. Also, estrogens do not cross-react to any significant degree with our anti-testosterone antibodies.

S. GROSS.   Your data are inadequate to conclude that immunologic specificity resides mainly in the A ring. Availability of functional determinants plays an important role. Because your conjugate blocks C-3 and/or C-17, you may be missing antibodies which can recognize these functional groups. It has been shown that a T-17 hapten cross-reacts less with a T-3 homolog than with a cortisone derivative blocked in the D ring. Finally, it is better to immunize with a steroid coupled to one large carrier and test with a non-cross-reacting carrier than to resort to absorption procedures.

A. SEHON.   One way of getting antibodies more specific for estrone or steroids in general would be for the organic chemist to synthesize smaller molecules which are part of the whole estrone molecule. In other words, start off with ring A, then ring B, and then attach to ring B a conjugating group and make antibodies to ring A plus ring B. In this way you limit your specificity from the beginning because you are going to stimulate antibody-forming cells which only recognize A and B. Then go on to A, B, D, C, or B and C, and C and D. In this way you are going to have various conformational parameters and antibodies formed against those specific regions of the molecule which might be exploited for a less heterogeneous population of antibodies, in the sense that the population would be more specific for the type of locus which you want to see.

L. GOODFRIEND.   Regarding the specificity of the aromatic ring: I think this is an important locus of specificity. We are dealing here with a region in which the A ring plays an important role. That more than the A ring is involved, however, was made evident in our turbidimetric studies by the inactivity of the dimethylphenols as hapten inhibitors in the interaction with antiserum to the C-17-estrone-protein conjugates. So it is not just the A ring that is involved in specificity; I think that a good deal, if not all, of the steroid backbone is also implicated.

J. TAIT.   What is the effect of lowering the temperature on the fluorescent interactions?

S. GROSS.   We have not looked at this yet. Ionic strength bears on the nature of binding.

E. GURPIDE.   To answer Dr. Fishman's previous question: The phenols do not compete with the anti-estriol antibodies. If you take a blank urine which contains phenol it is negative.

PART II
The Use of Antibodies for Radioimmunoassay of Steroid Hormones

4

PREPARATION AND PURIFICATION OF ANTIBODIES TO STEROIDS

Ian H. Thorneycroft,* Stephen A. Tillson, Guy E. Abraham,†
Rex J. Scaramuzzi, and Burton V. Caldwell

Worcester Foundation for Experimental Biology
Shrewsbury, Massachusetts

INTRODUCTION

As discussed in previous papers at this symposium, steroids or other low-molecular-weight compounds are not inherently antigenic (Goodfriend and Sehon, 1970; and Gross, 1970). Landsteiner, however, demonstrated in the early 1900's that antibodies directed against these low-molecular-weight compounds can be produced if they are chemically conjugated to a substance which is antigenic (see Landsteiner, 1946, for review). When conjugated to the antigen, these low-molecular-weight substances function as haptens.

Various steroid-protein conjugates have been prepared. The protein (antigen) has usually been either bovine serum albumin (BSA) or human serum albumin (HSA). To our knowledge antibodies to steroids were first reported by Sachs et al. (1925), and Sachs and Klopstock (1925). These authors mixed either lecithin or cholesterol with pig

* Present Address: Department of Obstetrics and Gynecology, University of Southern California, School of Medicine, 1321 N. Mission Road, Los Angeles, California 90033
† Present Address: Division of Endocrinology, Harbor General Hospital, Torrance, California.
This work was supported by training grant 5–T01–AMO 5564–13 from the National Institute of Arthritis and Metabolic Diseases, U.S.P.H.S., administered by Dr. Fernand G. Péron.

serum and obtained antibodies to these compounds. Von Mooser and Grilichess (1941) tried unsuccessfully to evoke antibodies to 5-androstene-3,7-diol by conjugating this compound in a *p*-amino-*O*-sulfobenzoate linkage to pig albumin, casein, and horse serum. Sprunt et al. (1951) published in abstract form that they had conjugated estradiol-17β to albumin of various species, and were able to produce antibodies to the steroid. The first comprehensive articles appearing on steroid antibodies were those from the group at Columbia University (Erlanger et al., 1957 and 1959; Beiser et al., 1959; and Lieberman et al., 1959) and the group at McGill University (Goodfriend and Sehon, 1958, 1960, 1961a and 1961b; and Goodfriend et al., 1961). The Columbia group synthesized oxime derivatives of steroidal ketone groups, using *o*-carboxymethylhydroxylamine (H₂NOCH₂COOH), and hemisuccinate or chlorocarbonate derivatives of steroid hydroxyl groups. The steroid derivatives were reacted, by the mixed anhydride method, with the free amino groups of BSA. The steroid-BSA conjugates when injected into rabbits elicited antibodies directed against the steroid haptens. The group from McGill prepared estrone-2-isocyanate and estrone-17-isocyanate and coupled these compounds to HSA to form either estrone-2-carbamido-HSA or estrone-17-carbamido-HSA. The details of these reactions have been discussed in a previous paper at this symposium (Goodfriend and Sehon, 1970). When injected into rabbits, these conjugates induced the formation of antibodies to estrone. Klopstock et al. (1964) synthesized cholesterol-3-formyl-BSA and cholanyl-24-BSA and successfully obtained antibodies to these şterols. Gross et al. (1968) prepared estradiol-17β-2- or 4-azobenzoic acid, coupled them to either BSA or KLH (keyhole limpet hemocyanin), and obtained antibodies of high specificity (Gross, 1970). There have been a number of other reports in recent years of success in obtaining antibodies to steroids, estradiol-17β in particular, but the methods employed have been basically the same as have been described above. A list of groups who have prepared antibodies to various steroids is given in Table 1.

For a complete review of the methods available to couple small molecules to antigens so they will function as haptens, there are the reviews by Beiser et al. (1968), Goodfriend and Sehon (1970), and Gross (1970).

The purpose of the studies to be reported here was to produce antibodies to steroids, estradiol-17β in particular, for use in a solid-phase radioimmunoassay.

In order for specific immunoglobulins directed against steroids to be practical for radioimmunoassay they should be (1) relatively easy to produce, (2) of high enough titer for widespread or long-term use, (3) sufficiently stable to allow either long-term storage or transportation, (4) as or more specific than the binding proteins from target tissues or

TABLE 1

Species and Conjugates Used for Immunization

Reference	Species immunized	Conjugate used
Sachs and Klopstock, 1925 Sachs et al., 1925	Rabbit	Cholesterol and lecithin mixed with pig serum
von Mooser and Grilichess, 1941	Rabbit	5-androstene-3,17-diol 3- or 17-p-amino-o-sulfo-benzoate conjugated to pig albumin, casein, and horse serum.
Sprunt et al., 1951	Rabbit	Estradiol-17β-albumin
Erlanger et al., 1957 and 1959 Beiser et al., 1959 Lieberman et al., 1959 Neri et al., 1964	Rabbit	Hemmisuccinate, chlorocarbonate and o-carboxymethyloxime derivatives of testosterone, progesterone, cortisone, cortisol, aldosterone, DOC, and estrone conjugated to BSA
Goodfriend and Sehon, 1958, 1960, 1961a and 1961b Goodfriend et al., 1961	Rabbit	Estrone-2 or 17-carbamido-HSA
Klopstock et al., 1964	Rabbit	Cholesterol-3-formyl-HSA and cholanyl-24-HSA
Zimmering et al., 1967	Sheep	Testosterone-17-formyl-BSA, and testosterone-3 or progesterone-20-o-carboxymethyloxime-BSA
Ferin et al., 1968	Sheep	Estradiol-17β-succinyl-BSA
Gross et al., 1968 Gross, 1970	Rabbit	Estradiol-17β 2- or 4-azobenzoyl-HSA or KLH
Jiang and Ryan, 1969	Rabbit	Estradiol-17β-succinyl-BSA
Midgley et al., 1969 Niswender and Midgley, 1970	Rabbit	Estradiol-17-formyl-BSA, and o-carboxymethyloxime, or hemisuccinate derivatives of testosterone, progesterone, estrone, estradiol, and 11-hydroxyprogesterone.
Tillson et al., 1970 Thorneycroft et al., 1970	Sheep and Rabbit	Testosterone-17-succinyl-BSA, progesterone 20-o-carboxymethyloxime-BSA and estradiol-17β-succinyl-BSA.

plasma, and (5) of high enough affinity to give greater sensitivity than presently available methods of steroid analysis. They must possess these characteristics in order to offer a superior technique to competitive protein binding using blood or target-tissue proteins. Neither of these latter two classes of specific proteins satisfies all five requirements listed above, and in many cases a ready or easy source of specific proteins is not available, e.g., aldosterone. This paper will discuss to what degree the immunoglobulins satisfy the first three requirements. The fourth and fifth will be discussed in other papers at this symposium (Abraham and Odell, 1970; Tillson et al., 1970; Niswender and Midgley, 1970; and Mikhail et al., 1970).

This paper will be divided into 5 sections:

1. Production of antibodies
2. Detection of antibodies
3. Rivanol purification of the antiserum
4. Titer and specificity of antibodies to estradiol evoked by two different BSA conjugates
5. Stability of gamma globulins

PRODUCTION OF ANTIBODIES

Sheep (N=4) and rabbits (N=4) were split into two equal groups. One group of each species was immunized with an estradiol-17β-succinyl-BSA conjugate [1,3,5(10)-estratriene-3,17β-diol, 17β-succinyl-BSA], and the second group with an estradiol-3-succinyl-BSA [1,3,5 (10) -estratriene-3,17β-diol, 3-succinyl-BSA]. The sheep were injected in multiple subcutaneous sites (near the axillary and pelvic lymph nodes) with 3 mg of estradiol-BSA conjugate dissolved in 5 ml of an emulsion of a 1:1 mixture of Freund's complete adjuvant and physiologic saline (0.9 percent NaCl). Each sheep received one injection per week for 6 weeks and monthly booster doses thereafter. All animals were bled 10 to 12 days after each booster. The rabbits were injected in multiple subcutaneous sites with 1 mg of conjugate in an emulsion of Freund's complete adjuvant and saline (1:1 mixture). They were injected once weekly for the first 6 weeks and then every 2 weeks for 4 months. Twelve days after the last immunization each animal was bled.

DETECTION OF ANTIBODIES

Detecting antibodies to steroid-protein conjugates is accomplished either by the basic immunologic techniques, such as the quantitative precipitin reaction or hemagglutination, or by comparing the ability of the antiserum proteins to bind the antigen or hapten more than serum from nonimmunized sheep. The precipitin test was used by Lieberman et al. (1959), Goodfriend and Sehon (1961a), Ferin et al. (1968), and Gross et al. (1968). Those papers concerned with developing antibodies for use in radioimmunoassay have generally employed the second technique. The antiserum is incubated with either the radioiodinated antigen (Midgley et al., 1969; and Niswender and Midgley, 1970), or the tritiated hapten (Abraham, 1969; Abraham and Odell, 1970; Jiang and Ryan, 1969; Tillson et al., 1970; and Mikhail et al., 1970), and the amount of labeled antigen or hapten bound to protein is measured. The many methods available for separating the bound and free antigen or hapten will be discussed in detail in other papers at this symposium (Tillson et al., 1970; Abraham and Odell, 1970; Niswender and Midgley, 1970; and Mikhail et al., 1970).

Animals injected with steroid-protein conjugates have been shown to manufacture antibodies to both the natural haptens of the protein and the steroids conjugated to them (Lieberman et al., 1959; Goodfriend and Sehon, 1961a; and Gross et al., 1968). Therefore, before a precipitin reaction can be run to detect and quantitate the anti-steroid titer, the antiserum must be adsorbed free of the anti-protein antibodies. Alternatively, one can run the precipitin reaction with a steroid-protein conjugate containing a protein not precipitated by the antibodies directed against the carrier protein. For example, if an animal is immunized with estradiol-BSA, then the precipitin reaction can be run with estradiol-HSA. The antigen must be used for the precipitin reaction as the free hapten will not form an insoluble complex with the antibody.

In this study each antiserum was adsorbed free of all anti-BSA antibodies for two reasons. First, to allow the investigator to run a precipitin reaction with the estradiol-BSA conjugate to detect and quantitate antibodies directed against estradiol*; and second, to remove unwanted antibodies, a process which is important in solid-phase radioimmunoassay and which will be discussed below.

To adsorb the antiserum free of anti-BSA antibodies, 0.5 ml of borate buffer (0.31 g boric acid, 0.50 g borax, 9.0 g NaCl in 1 liter H_2O) containing 5, 1, 0.5, 0.1, 0.05, or 0.01 mg of BSA was added to a series of glass tubes containing 0.5 ml of antiserum. The tubes were mixed and incubated at 37°C for 1 hour, followed by 48 hours incubation at 4°C. At the end of the incubation, the tubes were centrifuged and the tube containing the most precipitate selected. The amount of BSA per ml of antiserum necessary to maximally precipitate all of the anti-BSA antibodies was then calculated. The appropriate amount of a 2 percent BSA solution in borate buffer was added to the remainder of the antiserum, incubated, and centrifuged as above. The antiserum is now adsorbed free of anti-BSA antibodies.

A precipitin reaction with estradiol-17β-succinyl-BSA was run on SLC-9A (an antiserum from a sheep immunized with this conjugate for nine months) to demonstrate that specific antibodies to steroids had been

---

* Unless otherwise stated, estradiol will refer to estradiol-17β [1,3,5 (10) -estratriene-3, 17β-diol].

produced by this animal. From 0.6 mg to 2 mg of estradiol-17β-succinyl-BSA was dissolved in 0.5 ml of borate buffer and added to tubes containing 0.5 ml of BSA-adsorbed antiserum. Each level was run in triplicate. The tubes were mixed, incubated, and centrifuged as described above for the BSA adsorption. The precipitate was washed three times with 1 ml of cold distilled water, dried in a vacuum oven at 30°C overnight, and weighed on a Mettler microbalance. The oven contained $CaCl_2$ as a desiccant. The results are shown in Figure 1. The maximum precipitate occurred when 1.0 mg of conjugate was added. Subtracting this value from the weight of the precipitate, 11.0 mg, gave a value of 10.0 mg of antibody per 0.5 ml of antiserum, or 20.0 mg of antibody per ml of antiserum. Therefore, a specific antibody to the estradiol-17β-hemisuccinate was produced. Control tubes with an equivalent amount of BSA had an almost undetectable amount of precipitate.

The alternate method of detecting the antibodies to estradiol is to measure the ability of the antiserum proteins to bind a constant amount of ^3H-estradiol more than serum from nonimmunized animals. There are many methods available to separate the estradiol bound to protein from that which is free. We used the solid-phase method of Catt and Tregear (1967) as applied to radioimmunoassay of estradiol by Abraham (1969). This separation system will be described in detail by other papers at this symposium (Tillson et al., 1970; and Abraham and Odell, 1970). Basically, however, the solid-phase system functions in the following manner. When a dilution of serum or antiserum is added to polystyrene test tubes, the proteins bind tightly to the wall of the tube. The serum is removed after an appropriate length of time; the tubes now coated with protein are washed three times with the assay buffer. The proteins bound to the test tube are not removed by the washing. A solution containing

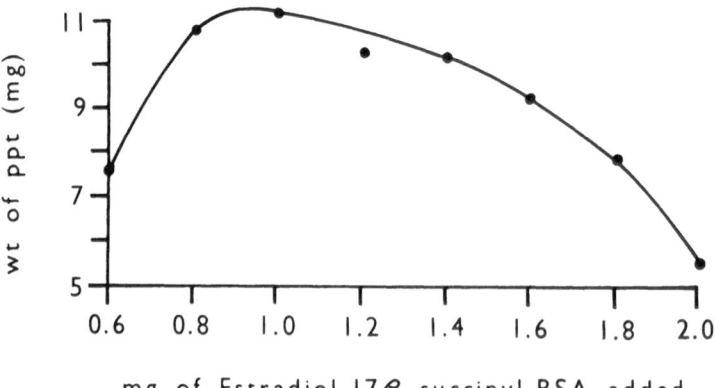

Fig. 1. A quantitative precipitin reaction for SLC-9A.

³H-estradiol is added to the protein coated tubes. After a further period of incubation the solution is withdrawn and counted. As this solution contains the hapten not bound by the serum proteins, the percent bound to the proteins can be calculated.

BSA-adsorbed antiserum (SLC-9A) was diluted 1:100, 1:500, 1:1,000, 1:5,000, 1:10,000, and 1:50,000. Serum from nonimmunized sheep was diluted 1:100, 1:500, and 1:1,000. Each dilution was accomplished using a sodium barbital buffer, pH 9.8 ($NaC_8H_{11}N_2O_3$, 7.2 g per 500 ml of distilled water). Aliquots of 0.4 ml of the diluted sera were pipetted into polystyrene test tubes and allowed to coat overnight at 4°C. The tubes were washed three times with 0.4 ml of a 0.1 M phosphate buffer (0.9 percent NaCl) pH 7.2. One-tenth of a milliliter of a solution of ³H-estradiol (40 c/mM) in phosphate buffer containing 0.05 µc per ml was added to each tube (0.005 µc per tube) and the volume brought up to 0.5 ml with phosphate buffer. The tubes were allowed to incubate at 4°C for 4 to 8 hours, after which the incubation medium was withdrawn, added to scintillation fluid, and counted (see Abraham and Odell, 1970, and Tillson et al., 1970, for further experimental details). The percent of the estradiol bound to protein was calculated and plotted as a function of dilution (Fig. 2). It is seen that the antiserum (SLC-9A) clearly bound more estradiol than the serum from nonimmunized sheep (solid line joined by dots and solid line joined by squares, respectively).

Titering an antiserum by measuring its ability to bind the antigen

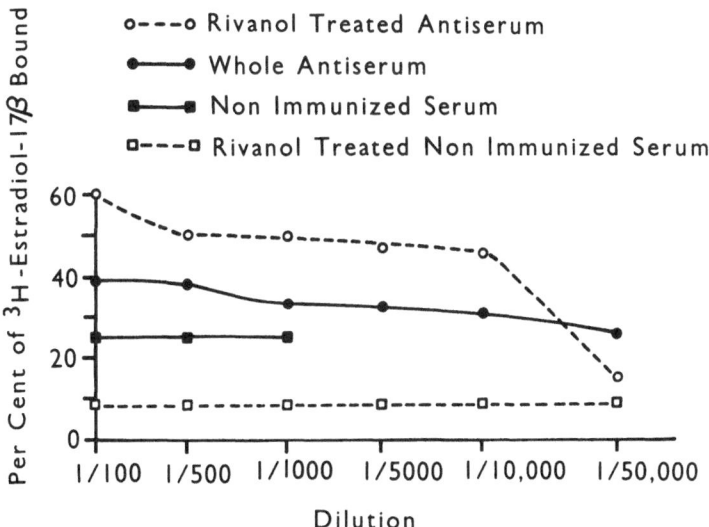

Fig. 2. The increase in hapten binding following Rivanol treatment of an antiserum (SLC-9A) in a solid-phase assay system.

or hapten is not the best method by immunologic criteria. However, it is the most relevant to radioimmunoassay, as the dilution curve tells the investigator if the serum binds and at what dilution the antiserum can be used for assay purposes.

To substantiate that the binding present in antiserum was indeed due to antibodies to estradiol, from 0 to 1.6 mg of estradiol-17β-succinyl-BSA was added to 0.5 ml aliquots of BSA-adsorbed antiserum (SLC-9A). The two were mixed, incubated, and centrifuged as described above. The supernatants were treated with Rivanol (see explanation in the next section), diluted 1:20 (final dilution of antiserum 1:100), and coated to plastic tubes. All coated tubes were incubated with ^{3}H-estradiol and the percent of steroid bound by the various supernatants calculated (Table 2). As increasing amounts of antigen were added the binding in the antiserum decreased. Between 0 and 1 mg of antigen represents the removal of the anti-estradiol antibodies; beyond 1 mg (the maximum precipitate point) (Fig. 1), the binding continued downward. Above 1 mg of antigen was the area of antigen excess, where a soluble antibody-antigen complex was formed. In this area the active sites of the antibody would be occupied by antigen molecules and hence would not be available for estradiol binding, resulting in lower binding. The fact that binding could be removed by precipitation with the antigen adds additional proof that the binding present in the antiserum was due to antibodies to estradiol. At the point of maximum precipitate there was 19.9 percent binding, 10 percent more than would be expected in normal nonimmunized sheep serum (Fig. 1., data after Rivanol treatment). All antibodies were not therefore removed by the precipitin reaction.

TABLE 2

Serum Binding of Estradiol-17β After Precipitation with Estradiol-17β-Succinyl-BSA

mg of estradiol-17β-succinyl-BSA added	Percent of ^{3}H-estradiol-17β bound by serum[a] after Rivanol treatment at pH 6.8
0.0	66.1
0.1	63.3
0.4	60.9
0.8	21.1
1.0	19.9
1.2	17.5
1.6	13.9

[a]The serum had previously been adsorbed free of all anti-BSA antibodies.

RIVANOL PURIFICATION OF THE ANTISERUM

In solid-phase systems not all of the protein added to the polystyrene test tubes is coated, only a certain percentage (Catt, 1969; and Tillson et al., 1970). Removing as many non-anti-estradiol gamma globulins and other blood proteins as possible should increase the number of anti-estradiol antibodies which become coated to the wall of the tube. Increased binding should result. All antisera were adsorbed free of the anti-BSA antibodies, as described above, in order to remove these unwanted gamma globulins.

Rivanol (2-ethoxy-6,9-diaminoacridine lactate) in 0.4 percent aqueous solution was reported by Horejsi and Smetana (1956) to precipitate all serum proteins, except gamma globulins, when added to serum (four parts of Rivanol solution to one part serum). Rivanol precipitation of proteins has been subsequently investigated and shown to be dependent on ionic strength of the buffer, concentration of Rivanol, and the pH of the solution (Tukachinskii and Moiseeva, 1961; Gurevich et al., 1961; and Neurath and Brunner, 1969). At pHs higher than a particular protein's isoelectric point, Rivanol forms an insoluble cationic complex with the protein.

Kaldor, Saifer, and Vecsler (1961) have investigated the mechanism of action of Rivanol precipitation of BSA and demonstrated that it is related to the number of carboxyl groups not interacting with amino groups. Rivanol has been used quite extensively in immunochemistry to obtain relatively pure gamma globulin preparations, which are, however, slightly contaminated with beta globulins. Styk et al. (1968) used Rivanol to remove nonspecific serum inhibitors of hemagglutination, and Prader et al. (1964) used it to demonstrate that the proteins used in an antiserum for radioimmunoassay were in fact gamma globulins. Abraham (1969) reported the use of Rivanol to purify antisera for use in solid-phase radioimmunoassay.

We have used Rivanol to purify our BSA-adsorbed antiserum. Antiserum (1 volume) was added to 4 volumes of an aqueous solution of Rivanol (0.4 percent), mixed, and allowed to stand at room temperature for 15 minutes, after which the solution was centrifuged and the supernatant decanted. The Rivanol left in the supernatant was removed by adding 200 mg of Norit A per 5 ml. The charcoal was removed by centrifugation. As a consequence of this procedure, the antiserum was diluted 1:5 and essentially devoid of all serum proteins except gamma globulins. Results of disc-gel electrophoresis, run by Miss Sheila Hunter of the Worcester Foundation, are illustrated in Figure 3. Rivanol precipitation under the above conditions removed most serum proteins, except gamma globulins and minute quantities of beta globulins.

Rivanol-treated and BSA-adsorbed antiserum (SLC-9A) and Rivanol-treated serum from nonimmunized sheep were diluted with barbital buffer to final dilutions of 1:100, 1:500, 1:1,000, 1:5,000, 1:10,000, and 1:50,000, and assayed for their estradiol binding activity in a solid-phase radioimmunoassay system as described above (Fig. 2). The binding in

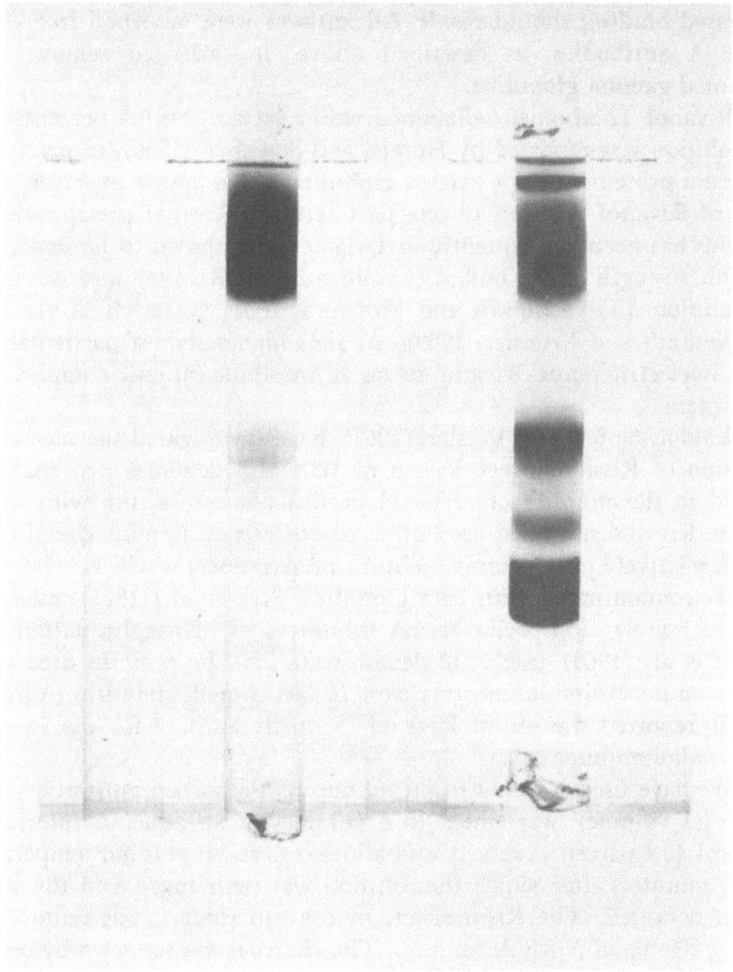

Fig. 3. Disc-gel electrophoresis of sera. On the right, sheep antiserum not treated with Rivanol. The characteristic protein bands are visible. From bottom to top: albumin, alpha globulin, beta globulin, and gamma globulin. On the left is an antiserum after Rivanol treatment. Gamma globulin and some beta globulin remain.

serum from nonimmunized sheep was reduced (compare dotted and solid lines joined by squares) and antiserum binding was increased (compare dotted and solid lines joined by circles). The hypothesis that removal of as many non-anti-estradiol proteins as possible would result in increased binding in solid-phase radioimmunoassay was confirmed.

If binding persists or increases in a solid-phase assay system after Rivanol treatment of the antisera, it would indicate that the binding was due to an immunoglobulin. Prader et al. (1964) used Rivanol to demonstrate binding by immunoglobulins.

Table 3 shows the effect of Rivanol precipitation on the dilution curves of two anti-estradiol antisera; in both cases Rivanol increased the specific binding.

The pH of the Rivanol solution is important. Figure 4 illustrates the effects of pH of the Rivanol on the binding of antiserum (SLC-9A) in a solid-phase radioimmunoassay. Binding increased as the pH increased until pH 8.8, after which binding decreased with an increase in pH. The increase up to pH 6 probably represented the removal of albumin, between 6 and 8 the removal of the alpha and beta globulins, and between 8 and 8.8 the removal of non-anti-estradiol gamma globulins. Above 8.8 the anti-estradiol gamma globulins were precipitated and the binding decreased. At pHs above 10.5 the Rivanol itself precipitates.

In a separate study, antisera treated with Rivanol at various pHs and antiserum not Rivanol-treated were electrophoresed on cellulose acetate at pH 8.6, and the percentage gamma globulins calculated. Concomitant Lowry protein determinations were run on all samples. The percentage of the gamma globulins remaining after Rivanol precipitation at var-

TABLE 3

The Effect of Rivanol[a] Treatment of Antisera on the Binding of Estradiol-17β to Anti-Estradiol in a Solid-Phase Radioimmunoassay

Serum dilution	Percent binding antiserum			
	SLC – 9A[b]		78 – 12D[c]	
	Without Rivanol	With Rivanol	Without Rivanol	With Rivanol
1:100	39.6	60.0	30.2	49.1
1:500	38.0	50.2	23.9	38.2
1:1,000	33.3	50.4	20.9	20.0
1:5,000	33.9	47.3	19.5	19.8
1:10,000	30.9	46.0	19.0	22.3
1:50,000	25.5	14.8	15.3	14.5

[a] 0.4% Aqueous solution, at pH 6.8.
[b] Immunized with estradiol-17-BSA.
[c] Immunized with estradiol-3-BSA.

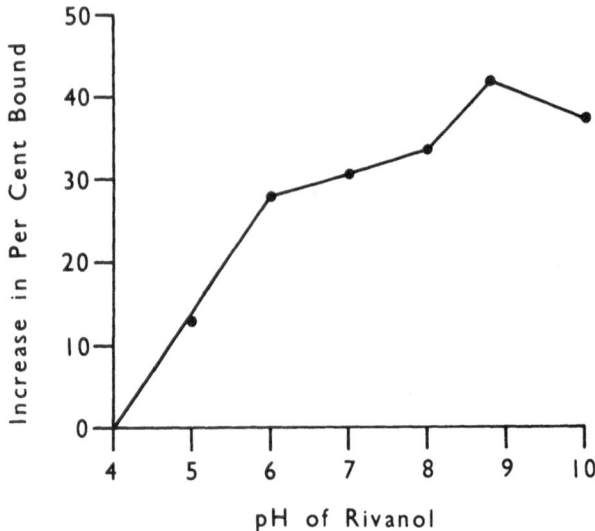

Fig. 4. The effect of changes in pH of Rivanol solution on the binding of estradiol to an antiserum. Increase in binding is expressed as a percent of the increase above that binding at pH 4.0 Rivanol solution.

ious dilutions was calculated. The assay titer of each was also calculated (Table 4). Higher pHs than we routinely used (6.8) would be indicated for sheep. Rabbits antisera, however, loses binding activity at pHs higher than 6.8 (Table 4). In the same table it is seen that sheep gamma globulins do not begin to precipitate until somewhere between pH 8.2 and 9.4.

TABLE 4

The Effect of pH of the Rivanol Solution on the Recovery of Gamma Globulins and on the Assay Titer of Anti-Estradiol in a Solid-Phase Radioimmunoassay

Species	pH	Percent of the gamma globulins not precipitated		Assay titer	
		Animal number		Animal number	
Rabbit		R-2	R-4	R-2	R-4
	6.8	84	76	1:2,000	1:1,000
	7.6	54	48	1:500	1:500
	8.4	36	38	1:100	1:100
Sheep					
	6.6	96		1:20,000	
	8.2	83		1:20,000	
	9.4	72		1:15,000	
	10.2	54		1:12,000	

This correlates well with the data in Figure 4 which indicated pH 8.8 as the most suitable pH. These data illustrate that each antiserum from each species must be checked for the pH of the Rivanol solution which gives optimum binding in a solid-phase radioimmunoassay system.

All results, unless otherwise stated, in the rest of this paper are on antisera which have been BSA-adsorbed and purified with Rivanol. The titer of the antibody for assay purposes will be called the "assay titer" and will refer to that dilution of antiserum which binds 45 to 50 percent of the labeled hapten added (30 to 60 pg). This is the most useful measure for radioimmunoassay purposes, as it tells one the dilution at which an antiserum can be used for assay purposes.

TITER AND SPECIFICITY OF ANTIBODIES TO ESTRADIOL EVOKED BY TWO DIFFERENT BSA CONJUGATES

Two different estradiol conjugates were used for immunization Table 5 reveals that in both sheep and rabbits better results were obtained with the 17-succinyl conjugate. The titers were much higher and there was 100 percent immunization success with this linkage. Only one animal (sheep 78) had a significant titer ($\geqq$1:100) after immunization with the 3-succinyl-conjugate. Aromatic esters are quite easy to saponify and the steroid residues of the 3-conjugate may have been cleaved off in vivo, resulting in a conjugate with fewer steroid residues,

TABLE 5

Comparison of the Anti-Estradiol Antibody Titer Induced by Different BSA-Estradiol Conjugates

Species	Estradiol-3-succinyl-BSA		Estradiol-17β-succinyl-BSA	
	Animal	Titer[a]	Animal	Titer
Rabbit	R-5	1:100 (5.5)[b]	R-1	1:500 (5.5)
	R-7	1:50 (5.5)[c]	R-3	1:500 (5.5)
Sheep	78	1:100 (12)	29	1:10,000 (10)
	86	0 (12)	SLC	1:20,000 (10)

[a]The titer is expressed as that dilution (after Rivanol treatment at pH 6.8) which binds 45 to 50% of 28 pg of ^{3}H-extradiol-17β.

[b]These animals had a maximum binding of 30% at the indicated dilutions.

[c]Number in parentheses represents the number of months immunized.

TABLE 6

Cross-Reaction of Estrone with Antibodies Evoked by Estradiol-BSA Conjugates

Species	Estradiol-3-succinyl-BSA		Estradiol-17β-succinyl-BSA	
	Animal	Cross-reaction %	Animal	Cross-reaction %
Rabbit	R-5	65 (5.5)[a]	R-1	38 (5.5)
	R-7	90 (5.5)	R-3	33 (5.5)
Sheep	78	50 (12)	SLC	33 (10)

[a] Number In parentheses represents the number of months immunized.

which could have rendered it less antigenic in producing antibodies to estradiol.

It was thought that the 3-position linkage would produce antibodies of higher specificity than the 17, as the 17-hydroxyl group would be unconjugated. This certainly was not the case as can be seen in Table 6. The cross-reaction with estrone was higher in those animals immunized with the 3 linkage. The percent cross-reaction is calculated in the same manner as reported by Abraham (1969). That is, cross-reaction is expressed in terms of the mass of unlabeled steroid which is required to displace 50 percent of the bound ^{3}H-estradiol.

Mass of estradiol required to displace 50 percent $= x$

Mass of cross-reacting steroid required for 50 percent

displacement $= y$

$(x/y) \ 100 =$ percent cross-reaction

It is difficult to explain why the 3 linkage did not produce more specific antibodies. Some in vivo oxidation of the 17-hydroxyl group may have occurred before the conjugate reached the site of antigen recognition.

Our experience would indicate, therefore, the 17β-succinyl-BSA linkage superior for estradiol immunizations, as higher titers and more specific antibodies were produced with this conjugate.

All animals were given many booster injections in an attempt to increase the assay titer. The reason for this was to obtain one antiserum which could be fully characterized and distributed to all interested investigators. The experience with polypeptide hormone radioimmunoassay has been that repeated immunizations reduced specificity. As an index of specificity each monthly bleeding of SLC was tested for cross-reaction with estrone (Fig. 5). Although the titer gradually increased from the fourth month on, the cross-reaction with estrone did not go up until the ninth month. Repeated immunizations were, therefore, warranted with this animal. We are currently assessing the results with 29, whose titer has also increased with time. Animal 78, whose titer went up several-fold

TABLE 7

Steroid Binding on Various Days after Immunization

Days after immunization	Percent binding antiserum	
	84-9[a]	SLC-6[b]
5	15.6	17.2
10	39.5	51.9
12	16.4	32.7
14	19.6	33.8
19	33.0	46.7

[a]Immunized against testosterone. Dilution of antiserum, 1:1,000.
[b]Immunized against estradiol-17β. Dilution of antiserum, 1:10,000.

between the eighth and twelfth months, had a 100 percent cross-reaction at 8 months and a 50 percent cross-reaction at 12 months. We have come to the conclusion that some form of chromatography step is necessary to separate the estrogens and, therefore, the increase in cross-reaction is not important.

The day of bleeding after immunization is important (Table 7). Animals should be bled at many different times after immunization to obtain peak (s) of antibody production. In the 78 animal, bleeding on various days after immunization meant obtaining an antiserum with a significant titer or not obtaining a titer at all.

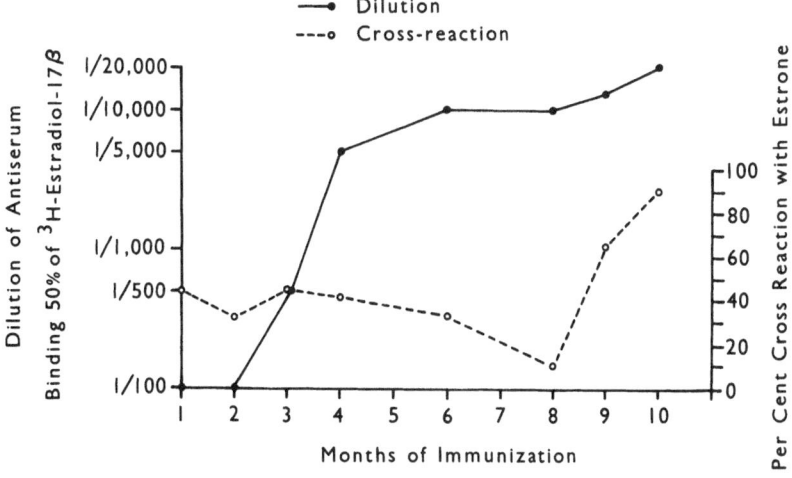

Fig. 5. The effect of repetitive immunizations on the binding of estradiol to an antiserum (SLC), and the corresponding cross-reaction with estrone.

TABLE 8

Effect of Repetitive Freezing and Thawing on Binding Activity of Anti-Estradiol Antibodies

Number of times frozen and thawed	Percent ^{3}H-estradiol bound to antiserum[a]	
	No Unlabeled Estradiol-17β Added	800 pg Unlabeled Estradiol-17β Added
1	30.7	9.4
5	31.8	10.9
10	30.7	10.3
15	32.6	12.3

[a]SLC-6X antiserum diluted 1:12,000.

TABLE 9

Stability of Antiserum with Time When Stored at Room Temperature

Time of storage (months)	Percent of ^{3}H-estradiol bound to antiserum[a]	
	No Unlabeled Estradiol-17β Added	400 pg Unlabeled Estradiol-17β Added
0	49.3	17.6
3	43.0	16.0

[a]SLC-6X antiserum diluted 1:10,000.

STABILITY OF GAMMA GLOBULINS

In our laboratory, the antibody is frozen in 10-ml aliquots of the Rivanol-treated material (1:5 dilution). One of these 10-ml bottles at a time is aliquoted into ten 1-ml aliquots and again frozen. To make up a solution for coating tubes, 0.1 ml of the 1:5 dilution is diluted to 1:10,000. The remaining solution is frozen again. A stock solution can, therefore, be frozen some 2 to 12 times before use. Table 8 shows that there was no effect of repetitive slow freezing and thawing on the binding and displacement of SLC-6X antiserum. Antisera have also been stored at −15°C for up to 1 year with no loss of binding activity. A sample of SCL-6X (which has sodium azide added) was left at room temperature for 3 months, with very little loss of binding activity (Table 9).

Acknowledgments

The authors wish to acknowledge Miss Miriam Kangas for technical assistance.

REFERENCES

Abraham, G. E. 1969. Solid-phase radioimmunoassay of estradiol-17β. J. Clin. Endocr., 29:866–870.

—— and W. Odell. 1970. Solid-phase radioimmunoassay of estrogens. *In* Péron, F. G., and B. V. Caldwell, eds. Immunologic Methods in Steroid Determination. New York, Appleton-Century-Crofts.

Beiser, S. M., B. Erlanger, F. Agate, and S. Lieberman. 1959. Antigenicity of steroid-protein conjugates. Science, 129:564–565.

—— V. P. Butler, Jr., and B. F. Erlanger. 1968. Hapten-protein conjugates: Methodology and application. *In* Miescher, P. A., and H. J. Muller-Eberhard, eds. Textbook of Immunopathology. Vol. 1, 15–52, New York, Grune & Stratton, Inc.

Catt, K. J. 1969. Solid phase separation systems. *In* M. Margaulies, ed. Protein and Polypeptide Hormones. Part 3, 639–642, New York, Excerpta Medica Foundation.

—— and G. W. Tregear. 1967. Solid-phase radioimmunoassay in antibody-coated tubes. Science, 158:1570–1572.

Erlanger, B. F., F. Borek, S. M. Beiser, and S. Lieberman. 1957. Steroid-protein conjugates. I. Preparation and characterization of conjugates of bovine serum albumin with testosterone and with cortisone. J. Biol. Chem., 228:713–727.

—— F. Borek, S. M. Beiser, and S. Lieberman. 1959. Steroid-protein conjugates. II. Preparation and characterization of conjugates of bovine serum albumin with progesterone, deoxycorticosterone, and estrone. J. Biol. Chem., 234:1090–1094.

Ferin, M., P. E. Zimmering, S. Lieberman, and R. L. Vande Wiele. 1968. Inactivation of the biological effects of exogenous and endogenous estrogens by antibodies to 17β-estradiol. Endocrinology, 83:565–571.

Goodfriend, L., and A. H. Sehon. 1958. Preparation of an estrone-protein conjugate. Canad. J. Biochem. Physiol., 36:1177–1184.

—— and A. H. Sehon. 1960. Antigenicity of oestrone-protein conjugates. Nature (London), 185:764–766.

—— and A. H. Sehon. 1961a. Antibodies to estrone-protein conjugates. I. Immunological studies. Canad. J. Biochem. Physiol., 39:941–960.

—— and A. H. Sehon. 1961b. Antibodies to estrone-protein conjugates. II. Endocrinological studies. Canad. J. Biochem. Physiol., 39:961–965.

—— and A. H. Sehon. 1970. Early approaches to production, analysis, and use of steroid antisera. *In* Péron, F. G., and B. V. Caldwell, eds. Immunologic Methods in Steroid Determination. New York, Appleton-Century-Crofts.

—— A. Leznoff, and A. H. Sehon. 1961. Antibodies to estrone-protein conjugates. III. Tissue localization of estrogens. Canad. J. Biochem. Physiol., 39:967–971.

Gross, S. J. 1970. Specificities of steroid antibodies. *In* Péron, F. G., and B. V. Caldwell, eds. Immunologic Methods in Steroid Determination. New York, Appleton-Century-Crofts.

—— D. H. Campbell, and H. H. Weethall. 1968. Production of antisera to steroids coupled to proteins directly through the phenolic A ring. Immunochemistry, 5:55–65.

Gurevich, A. E., M. Gubernieva, and K. N. Myasoedova. 1961. A comparison of the enzymatic hydrolyzates of non-specific gamma globulins and antibodies of rabbits. Biochemistry (USSR), 26: 413–422.

Horejsi, J., and R. Smetana. 1956. The isolation of gamma globulin from blood-serum by Rivanol. Acta Med. Scand., 155:65–70.

Jiang, N. S., and R. J. Ryan. 1969. Radioimmunoassay for estrogens: A preliminary communication. Mayo Clin. Proc., 44:461–465.

Kaldor, G., A. Saifer, and F. Vecsler. 1961. The interaction of Rivanol with BSA. Arch. Biochem., 94:207–216.

Klopstock, A., M. Pinto, and A. Rimon. 1964. Antibodies reacting with steroid haptens. J. Immun., 92:515–519.

Landsteiner, K. 1946. Specificity of Serological Reactions. Cambridge, Mass., Harvard University Press.

Lieberman, S., B. F. Erlanger, S. M. Bieser, and F. J. Agate, Jr. 1959. Steroid-protein conjugates: Their chemical, immunochemical, and endocrinological properties. Recent Progr. Hormone Res., 15:165–200.

Midgley, A. R., Jr., G. D. Niswender, and J. S. Ram. 1969. Hapten-radioimmunoassay: A general procedure for the estimation of steroidal and other haptenic substances. Steroids, 13:731–737.

Mikhail, G., M. Ferin, and R. L. Vande Wiele. 1970. Radioimmunoassay of estrogens by polymerization. *In* Péron, F. G., and B. V. Caldwell, eds. Immunologic Methods in Steroid Determination. New York, Appleton-Century-Crofts.

Mooser, H., and R. K. Grilichess. 1941. Immunisierungsversuche mit Steroiden. Schweiz. Z. allgem. Pathol. u. Bakteriol., 4:375–380.

Neri, R. O., S. Tolksdorf, S. M. Beiser, B. F. Erlanger, F. J. Agate, Jr., and S. Lieberman. 1964. Further studies on the biological effects of passive immunization with antibodies to steroid-protein conjugates. Endocrinology, 74:593–598.

Neurath, A. R., and R. Brunner. 1969. Fractionation of proteins with different isoelectric points by Rivanol. Experientia, 25:668–671.

Niswender, G. D., and A. R. Midgley, Jr. 1970. Hapten-radioimmunoassay of steroid hormones. *In* Péron, F. G., and B. V. Caldwell, eds. Immunologic Methods in Steroid Determination. New York, Appleton-Century-Crofts.

Prader, A., H. Wagner, J. Szeky, R. Illig, J. L. Touber, and D. Maingay. 1964. Acquired resistance to human growth hormone caused by specific antibodies. Lancet, 2:378–382.

Sachs, H., and A. Klopstock. 1925. Die serologische Differenzierung von Lecithin und Cholesterin. Biochem. Z., 159:491–501.

—— A. Klopstock, and A. J. Weil. 1925. Die Entstehung der syphilitischen Blutveraenderung, Deutsch. Med. Wschr., 51:589–592.

Sprunt, D. H., A. D. Dulaney, and R. Conger. 1951. Methods of preparation and antigenic activity of estrogen-protein conjugates. Cancer Res., 11:282.

Styk, B., N. J. Schmidt, and J. Dennis. 1968. The use of Rivanol treatment for removal from sera of non-specific inhibitors of enterovirus and reovirus hemagglutination. Amer. J. Epidem., 88:398–405.

Tukachinskii, S. E., and V. P. Moiseeva. 1961. Binding of Rivanol with serum proteins. Biochemistry (USSR), 26:104–108.

Tillson, S. A., I. H. Thorneycroft, G. E. Abraham, and B. V. Caldwell. 1970. Solid-phase radioimmunoassay of steroids. *In* Péron, F. G., and B. V. Caldwell, eds. Immunologic Methods in Steroid Determination. New York, Appleton-Century-Crofts.

Zimmering, P. S., S. Lieberman, and B. Erlanger. 1967. Binding of steroids to steroid-specific antibodies. Biochemistry (Wash.), 6:154–164.

DISCUSSION

D. PRESSMAN.   You pointed out that there would be an advantage in using a different carrier protein to test for antisteroid activity. I wonder why you precipitate the anti-BSA antibodies with added BSA before carrying our your test; because in your test, you really do not care whether you have some anti-BSA antibodies or any other kind of antibodies. You are concerned only with the anti-steroid antibodies.

I. THORNEYCROFT.   The reason we adsorb the serum free of anti-BSA antibodies is to allow more estradiol-specific antibodies to bind to the plastic tubes. There is only a fixed number of sites on the plastic tubes. Therefore, by removing unwanted proteins, more specific proteins should be bound.

D. PRESSMAN.   Yes, but as long as you have so much normal globulin present, a little bit of anti-BSA is not going to interfere. I think it is an extra step which is not necessary if you are using your binding on the tubes as the test.

I. THORNEYCROFT.   It is only really necessary if there is a high titer of anti-BSA antibodies.

G. ABRAHAM.   The titer of anti-BSA goes as high as 20 mg/ml. If we do not remove the anti-BSA we are not giving the anti-estrogen antibody a chance to coat the tube.

A. SEHON.   If you really want to get rid of any extraneous proteins in order to increase the amount of specific antibodies bound to the walls of the test tubes, the simplest thing would be to use some immuno-absorbent.

G. ABRAHAM.   That is beautiful theoretically, but the immuno-absorbent does not work for high-affinity antibodies. You just cannot remove them from the immuno-adsorbent once they have been absorbed. We have tried high-ionic strength, low pH, and blessed water and were not successful. It is very nice to adsorb antibodies, but you must also remove them and this we could not do.

A. SEHON.   I realize that high-affinity antibodies may stick tenaciously to your immuno-solvent; however, you have indicated in the slides that with an addition of 800 pg of estradiol you are displacing the tritiated material. If you displace it, it means that you have an irreversible reaction. Therefore you either measure the very weakly bound estradiol on displacement, or the reaction is not irreversible and you can reverse it.

I. THORNEYCROFT.   Yes, it is true that the binding is reversible. However, Dr. Burstein in his paper will show that adding micrograms of estradiol did not seem to displace the protein from the immuno-absorbent.

S. GROSS.   Steroid antibody molecules resist acid dissociation, probably because of potent hydrophobic interaction. It seems reasonable that the yield would be improved by the use of urea. Reactivity of recovered protein may be diminished. How many milligrams of IgG is present in sheep serum?

I. THORNEYCROFT.   There is ordinarily about 11 mg/ml.

S. GROSS.   And yet you brought down 20 mg/ml of antibody with a small amount of antigen? I wonder what the valence of the antibody was calculated to be?

I. THORNEYCROFT.   It was not calculated, but is probably quite high.

S. GROSS.   Certainly not two.

I. THORNEYCROFT.   Correct.

S. GROSS.   I am worried about this antibody. Perhaps some of it is still directed to the carrier protein.

I. THORNEYCROFT.   The 20 mg of antibody bothered us, as it is twice the normal amount of gamma globulin. One ml of BSA-adsorbed SLC-9A and 1 ml of serum from a nonimmunized animal were Rivanol-treated, and Lowry protein analyses were performed on the supernatant. SLC-9A had 31 mg/ml of protein and normal serum 11 mg. There was certainly enough gamma globulin in the immunized animal to account for the 20 mg of anti-estradiol. In fact, the difference in total gamma globulin between normal and immunized animals was 20 mg, exactly equal to the figure determined by the precipitin reaction. SLC appears from electrophoretic studies to have compensated by reducing albumin. It must also be pointed out that SLC is a hyperimmunized animal, having been immunized for 9 months.

Another interesting fact about SLC is her hematocrit, which has been 20 percent for some 4 or 5 months; the normal value is about 45 percent.

Regarding your question about the completeness of the BSA-adsorption, a second precipitin reaction with BSA revealed no detectable titer.

L. GOODFRIEND.   You obviously have a highly hyperimmunized animal in which a good deal of the gamma globulin is antibody. It seems to me that you have here a nice opportunity to see what kind of cross-reactions you get with other steroids. Do you have any data concerning this?

I. THORNEYCROFT.   We have only characterized one bleeding fully, the SLC-6X. Dr. Tillson will be giving the full details of that antiserum. Essentially, the only cross-reaction after 6 months of immunization was with the estrogens; estrone, estradiol-17α, and a low cross-reaction with estriol. Other steroids did not cross-react at all. Cross-reaction studies have not been run on the ninth bleeding (the one on which the precipitin reaction was reported; see Chap. 4, Fig. 1). I would, however, suspect that the cross-reaction with testosterone may indeed have gone up, because the cross-reaction with estrone had gone up from 33 to 65 percent between the sixth and ninth months.

G. NISWENDER.   I would like to substantiate that to which Dr. Abraham has referred. In our laboratory we have also tried immuno-absorbents. We have tried varying pH from 12 to 1. We have tried acetic acid and hydrochloric acid buffers, as well as high and low temperatures. We have tried to elute antibodies within 10 minutes of the initial binding reaction and have never been able to demonstrate a single recoverable antibody from this kind of an experiment. In addition, we have added tremendous excesses of cold estradiol and, again, we cannot recover a single antibody with the techniques which we have been using. I think this brings us to another very interesting point about these curves. I am not sure that these are really dose-response curves. I wonder, Dr. Thorneycroft, have you ever added the radioactive hormone and the cold hormone to these assay tubes in a nonequilibrium condition? In other words, have you ever added radioactive hormone first and then cold hormone and, if so, do you get a dose-response curve?

I. THORNEYCROFT.   No, the routine assay that we perform is that of Dr. Abraham, in which both the radioactive and cold hormone are added together.

G. NISWENDER.   We have done these experiments and found that, even with the protein hormones, at least in most of the systems in our laboratory, one does not displace with the hot hormone. In fact, the first antigen which is bound to the antibody apparently is bound irreversibly and the only thing the hot hormone combines with is unoccupied sites that are remaining. This apparently is true for the proteins in the systems we have checked and also for the steroids. In other words, if we add the hot hormone first and then varying quantities of standard cold hormone, we do not get a dose-response curve.

You have suggested that, in at least two rabbits, when you immunized with a 17 derivative rather than a 3 derivative of estrone you reduce the cross-reaction from 65 to 38 percent. I wonder if you think that, in two rabbits, this extent of reduction has any physiologic meaning or if this could be merely differences between rabbits instead of differences between the structure of the antigen.

I. THORNEYCROFT. Yes, it could quite well be. There is a possibility, I don't know if you would like to comment on it, that there may be some in vivo conversion of the 3 conjugate; that is, oxidation of estradiol to estrone. I am sure that no one has checked this out.

Dr. Sehon mentioned earlier that column purification would be a superior technique for antibody purification for use in solid-phase radio-immunoassay. We have tried another method of purification. The anti-estradiol antibody was precipitated with the optimum mass of estradiol-17β-succinyl-BSA. The precipitate was washed and then dissolved in water whose pH had been adjusted with HCl to 2.5. It was theorized that under these conditions, the antigen and antibody would be dissociated and that if this solution were then Rivanol treated, in the manner described in this paper, then the BSA-estradiol conjugate would precipitate, leaving the antibody in solution. The pH 2.5 solution of the antibody and antigen was Rivanol-treated (final pH 5.0), the supernatant diluted 1:20 (1:100 final dilution) and coated to polystyrene test tubes. Figure 1 illustrates that the whole antiserum at a 1:100 dilution bound 40 percent and following Rivanol treatment bound 60 percent. Antisera purified by dissolving the precipitate bound 90 percent at a 1:100 dilution, further demonstrating that antiserum purification increases binding, due to more specific proteins occupying the fixed number of binding sites on the polystyrene test tubes (Abraham and Odell, 1970). Unfortunately, we have been unable to duplicate this purification procedure. Apparently, when the pH adjusts back to the pH at which the antigen and antibody become tightly bound, the Rivanol does nothing but precipitate antibody-antigen complex with no protein remaining in solution.

P. ZIMMERING. I just wanted to add some information about our experience with hyperimmunized sheep. We found in 12 different sheep, using five different steroid conjugates, that the animals did develop very high amounts of gamma globulin, not all of which were antibodies to these steroid conjugates. These were very high-titered animals. The electrophoretic patterns were completely reversed from what one usually sees, with very high gamma globulin peaks and even normal albumin peaks. The albumin did not seem to be reduced, although we did not measure it. One animal with over 80 mg of antibody per ml survived for quite a long time, however.

W. D. ODELL.   One of the general questions of a practical nature which one would hope to come out of a workshop like this is: What species of animal is the best for immunization with steroid conjugates? My general impression, which emerges from the published papers and also from conversations with a variety of people, is that sheep may be preferable. If possible, however, I would like to have us collect some objective data on this. Could you give us your total experience on all numbers of animals immunized and a rough impression of their results, or do the two rabbits and the two sheep immunized with each conjugate represent the total experience?

I. THORNEYCROFT.   Yes, I reported all of our immunizations.

R. ZIMMERING.   We did both rabbits and sheep but we never ran our rabbits up to that area by titer. Most of the work was done on the comparative binding, and binding constants were from sheep antibody.

W. D. ODELL.   Obviously, if specificity is the problem, then small animals in large numbers would be the proper way to develop antisera. If titer is the problem and specificity is not, then larger animals and large volumes of blood would be advantageous.

I. THORNEYCROFT.   We have concluded that some form of chromatography will be necessary in steroid radioimmunoassay. The cross-reaction, particularly with estrone, is not very troublesome, as the antiserum can be used for both the assay of estrone and of estradiol if a chromatographic separation is employed.

A. GROSSBERG.   In the solid-phase assay, if you have high-binding antibodies and decrease the amount of estrone you are using, you should get essentially 100 percent binding of the ligand. Have you observed this?

G. ABRAHAM.   It is true that, theoretically, we should get 100 percent binding at high concentration of antibody with regard to the hapten, but when one considers some thermodynamic conditions, we find that we are using a dilution of antibodies and hapten which is sometimes two powers lower than the affinity constant of the antiserum. One would expect under those conditions that not all the sites would be saturated—even less than 50 percent of them.

A. MIDGLEY.   If one examines the curves concerning Rivanol-treated and non-treated sera, you reached a plateau and the plateau continued as the antibody concentration was increased. My interpretation would be that there was a higher effective concentration. Since there is a plateau, I would think that the limitation here is probably one of time. If you were to incubate for a much longer time you could take advantage of the high-affinity constant and might get a higher percent binding. However, I think this argument could cause some difficulty. As you dilute the antiserum out, you finally reach a point where there is no difference between Rivanol-treated and non-Rivanol-treated serum in terms of the binding.

I. THORNEYCROFT. We have found prolonged incubation does not increase the binding greatly. The limiting factor is how much mass of protein becomes coated to the polystyrene test tube.

A. MIDGLEY. Regarding the prolonged incubation one does not get any higher amount of binding. It is surprising that there are these differences in plateaus because it represents excess antibody in both cases unless the presence of nonimmune globulin is blocking the sites.

I. THORNEYCROFT. It is true that there is an excess of antibody in the plateau regions (see Chap. 4, Fig. 3) of both the whole antiserum and the Rivanol-treated antiserum. However, since the Rivanol-treated antiserum contains a greater percentage of anti-estradiol antibodies than the whole antiserum, and since only a certain percentage of all proteins coat to the tubes, the Rivanol-purified preparation should coat more specific antibodies to the wall of the test tube, hence increase binding.

A. MIDGLEY. Dr. Thorneycroft, you are making quite a distinction between the 3 and 17 derivative of the estradiol. I believe these were succinyl derivatives. If you make these comparisons, do you have physicochemical data to indicate that the materials used as antigens are indeed comparable, that is, that it is simply a 3 derivative and not a 3, 17, and that the number of residues of estradiol per protein molecule are comparable, and therefore that the sheep and rabbits were immunized with comparable amounts of determinant sites?

I. THORNEYCROFT. The conjugates were obtained from Dr. Abraham. I think he should answer your question.

G. ABRAHAM. In 3-position conjugation, only a short incubation with succinic anhydride and pyridine was required because the 3-phenolic hydroxyl was more reactive than the 17 hydroxyl. However, to prepare the 17 conjugate, one had first to prepare the disuccinate, then split the 3 position with potassium hydroxide and methanol. We have not purified the succinate derivative very extensively, and there might have been some of the disuccinate in the 17 conjugate. We felt we did not need such high purity since the sheep were going to respond to about 20 different haptens and adding one at the 3 position would not make much difference. We were interested in removing from the complex the one antibody of particular interest to us. We did add tritiated estradiol to the cold estradiol to calculate the amount of incorporation of estradiol into the protein. There were 17 steroids per BSA molecule when the 3-succinate was used, and 23 when the 17-succinate was used.

5

SOLID-PHASE RADIOIMMUNOASSAY OF SERUM ESTRADIOL-17β: A SEMI-AUTOMATED APPROACH

G. E. Abraham and W. D. Odell

Division of Endocrinology, Harbor General Hospital
Torrance, California

INTRODUCTION

Estrogens, like other steroids, exist in the organism in many forms, the predominant form depending on the particular biologic fluid. In urine, estrogens are almost entirely in the conjugated forms, as sulfates, β-glucuronides, and other less common conjugates. In blood, however, a significant proportion of the estrogens exist in the free (unconjugated) form. Both free and conjugated estrogens can be bound to intra- and extracellular proteins. It is beyond the scope of this presentation to expand further on this aspect of estrogen metabolism. (For review on above subjects, see Preedy, 1968). However, it must be emphasized that a comprehensive study of estrogen metabolism is a formidable task, in view of the large number of estrogens found in biologic materials and the various forms in which they exist.

An alternative is to limit oneself to one or a few estrogens in one form, in one biologic fluid. Factors that will decide which estrogens to measure include the kind of study to be undertaken and the methods available. In physiologic studies, attention is usually directed toward the most potent estrogen known, estradiol-17β (hereafter referred to as E_2). Although there are many physicochemical methods for the detection of

Supported by USPHS grants AM-5550 and 5-ROI-HD02701.

E_2 (Preedy, 1968), none of them has been shown to be sufficiently specific for quantitative estimation in biologic fluids without extensive purification and separation of E_2 from interfering materials.

Recently, another detection method has been applied successfully to the estimation of free (unconjugated) steroids in blood. In this approach, termed radioimmunoassay by Berson and Yalow (1959), saturation analysis by Ekins (1960), competitive protein-binding radioassay by Murphy (1964), and radioligand binding assay (when applied to steroids) by Korenman et al. (1969), a compound to be measured is allowed to compete with a similar or a chemically related radioactive compound for a limited number of binding sites on specific binding proteins. Table 1 shows some possible sources of binding reagents used in this approach. The free and bound labeled compounds are separated by various means (Table 2). Afterwards, the partition of the labeled compounds between the free and bound fractions is evaluated, and since this is a function of the mass of the unlabeled compounds present, the mass of these compounds in unknown samples can be calculated by interpolation on a standard curve.

We have recently reported an assay procedure for E_2 (Abraham, 1969) based on the principles described above, using an antibody preparation as a specific binding reagent, obtained by active immunization of a ewe for 15 months with estradiol-17β-hemisuccinate-bovine serum albumin conjugate. This antiserum reacted only with naturally occurring estrogens, and more so with E_2 than any other estrogen tested. A solid-phase system was chosen to separate free from bound labeled hormones. When this detection method was applied to the determination of E_2 in the dried ether extract of plasma samples, it was found not to be completely specific for E_2 when low levels of E_2 were present. We have since

TABLE 1

Sources of Specific Proteins Used in the Competitive-Protein Binding Radioassay

I. Intracellular
    A. Uterine Cytosol (Rabbit, Sheep)

II. Extracellular
    A. Plasma Binding Proteins
        1. Thyroxin binding globulins
        2. Transcortin
        3. Testosterone, 5 α-dihydro-testosterone, estradiol-17β-binding proteins
    B. Immunoglobulins
        1. Ig M
        2. Ig A
        3. Ig G

TABLE 2

Available Methods for Separation of Free from Bound Hormone

I. Chromatographic
   - A. Paper
   - B. Cellulose Column
   - C. Sephadex Column

II. Precipitation of Bound Form
   - A. Salt
   - B. Alcohol
   - C. Ammonium Sulfate
   - D. Dioxane
   - E. Double Antibody

III. Precipitation of Free Form
   - A. Dextran Coated Charcoal
   - B. Ion-exchange Resin
   - C. Precipitated Silica

IV. Solid-Phase System
   - A. Cellulose-antibody Complex
   - B. Sephadex-antibody Complex
   - C. Polystyrene-antibody Complex
   - D. Antibody-coated Polystyrene Tube

incorporated in the assay a rapid chromatographic system, capable of separating all the known interfering estrogens except estradiol-17α. With this purification step, the detection method used was found to be specific for plasma E_2.

A detailed description of this method will be presented, the reagents characterized, and the results obtained when tested for reliability and practicability discussed.

MATERIALS

Solvents

Diethylether (Mallinkrodt AR anhydrous) was obtained in 1-lb cans and stored at $-20°C$. A freshly opened can was used for the plasma extraction. The cold ether was transferred into an Oxford pipettor P-5058-2 (Standard Products, Los Angeles, Calif.) and placed into a melting ice bath. After use, the ether was discarded. Isooctane, ethylene glycol, and ethyl acetate were obtained from Matheson, Coleman and Bell (Los Angeles, Calif.) in spectrograde quality. Once a bottle of solvent was opened, the solvent blank gradually rose with time. The greatest effect on the blank was produced by ethyl acetate. It is recommended, therefore, that all solvents be stored in small aliquots, tightly closed and used a few times only. If the dried residue of 5 ml of a solvent gave a blank equivalent to more than 20 pg of E_2, this batch of solvent was not used in the assay.

Buffers

BUFFER FOR COATING.   Barbital buffer (the sodium salt) at a concentration of 0.07 M in deionized, distilled water was used to dilute the partially purified antiserum prior to coating the plastic tubes, as described later. Sodium azide was added at a concentration of 1 mg/ml to prevent bacterial and mold growth. The unadjusted pH was usually 9.6 with a range of 9.5 to 9.7. When we attempted to adjust the pH with NaOH or HCl, the resulting buffer gave poor results when used to coat the plastic tubes with the antibody preparation; low binding of $^3H\text{-}E_2$ and marked variations in binding of $^3H\text{-}E_2$ from tube to tube were noted. It was later found that the quality of the water used to prepare the buffer affected the final pH and in some instances the unadjusted pH of the buffer was as low as 8.2. We therefore used freshly deionized, glass-distilled water throughout the assay. Barbital buffer was prepared fresh monthly and kept at 4°C. Even under these conditions, occasional mold growth occurred. Prior to use, the bottle containing this buffer was shaken gently, and if it appeared slightly cloudy with evidence of mold growth, it was discarded. This buffer will hereafter be referred to as coating buffer.

BUFFER FOR ASSAY.   The buffer used in the assay procedure was exactly as described previously (Abraham, 1969). A detailed description of its preparation is as follows:

Two stock solutions of sodium phosphate buffer, 0.2 M, were prepared:

Solution A=27.6 g $NaH_2PO_4 \cdot H_2O$/liter H_2O
Solution B = 53.65 g $Na_2HPO_4 \cdot 7H_2O$/liter H_2O

The assay buffer was prepared by adding to a 1-liter bottle:

195 ml of solution A
305 ml of solution B
1 g of sodium azide
9 g of sodium chloride
500 ml of water

It was kept at room temperature with a shelf life of about 1 month. The unadjusted pH was usually 7.0 with a range of 6.9 to 7.1. The quality of the water used was of utmost importance in obtaining this unadjusted pH. This buffer will hereafter be referred to as assay buffer.

Radioisotopically Labeled E₂

γ-EMITTING ISOTOPES. E_2 may be labeled with radioisotopes emitting β-
or γ-radiations. Because of the phenolic ring A, radioactive halogens such
as ^{82}Br, ^{125}I, and ^{131}I may be incorporated into the ring A at the positions
C-2 and C-4 (Fig. 1). However, ^{82}Br has a short half-life which limits its

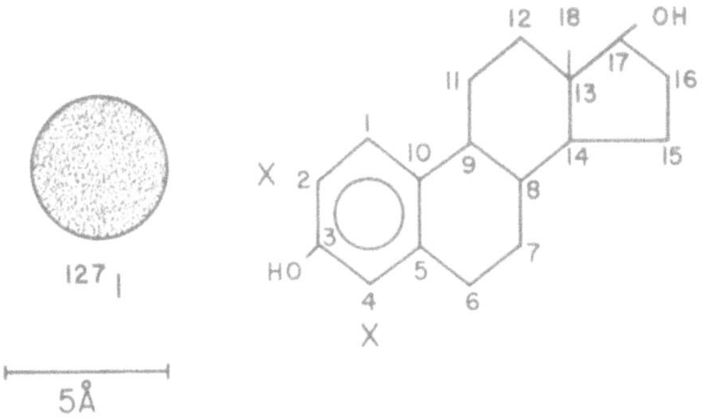

Fig. 1. Schematic representation of the relative sizes of an atom of ^{127}I and a
molecule of E_2. "X" represents the sites of halogenation.

use to a few days only. The same limitation, although to a lesser extent,
applies to ^{125}I and ^{131}I. Another factor that almost rules out the radioactive halogens as a possible marker on the E_2 molecule is inherent in
their physical properties. First, they are highly electronegative atoms and
significantly affect the net charge of the molecules into which they are
incorporated. Secondly, the radioactive halogens with the longest half-life
are relatively large atoms and would interfere with the steric fitness of the
antibody active sites. For instance, the iodine atom is larger than ring
A of E_2. (The van der Waals' radii are, respectively: $^{127}I = 2.15$ Å;
benzene $= 1.70$Å.) (Pressman and Grossberg, 1968).

β-EMITTING ISOTOPES. E_2 is commercially available, labeled with ^3H or
^{14}C. Although these β-emitters have specific activities several orders of
magnitude lower than the γ-emitters, they are nevertheless adequate for
the present purpose.

Tritium has a greater specific activity than ^{14}C because of its shorter
half-life. 6,7 ^3H-E_2 is available with specific activities ranging from 40
to 50 curies/mM (New England Nuclear, Boston, Mass.). More recently,
2,4,6,7 ^3H-E_2 has become commercially available with a specific activity
of 100 curies/mM (Amersham-Searle, Chicago, Ill.). However, the tritium
atoms at the C-2 and C-4 positions of E_2 appeared to interfere with
binding to the anti-E_2 preparation, as will be shown later. For this reason,
6,7 ^3H-E_2 was chosen for use in the assay procedure. It was received from
the supplier in benzene:ethanol (9:1) and was stored at 4°C in the same

solvent mixture at a concentration of 20 μc/ml. There was no evidence of damage after up to 3 months of storage. The radioactive tracer was replaced every 3 months.

E_2 Standard

E_2 was obtained from Sigma Chemical Corporation (St. Louis, Mo.) in the purest form available. A solution in absolute ethanol was prepared containing 100 ng/ml and stored at —20°C in 0.5-ml aliquots. For each assay, an aliquot was warmed to room temperature and 0.1 ml was added to a glass vial and dried. Ten milliliters of assay buffer was added to dissolve the dried residue. This solution contained 1 pg of E_2/μl of buffer and was used for the standard curve.

Antibody Preparation

The preparation and purification of the antiserum used have been previously described (Abraham, 1969). For purification, 1 ml of antiserum was mixed with 4 ml of an aqueous solution of 0.4 percent Rivanol at a pH of 6.8. Albumin and α-globulins were not found when the purified antiserum was electrophoresed on cellulose acetate strips (Fig. 2).

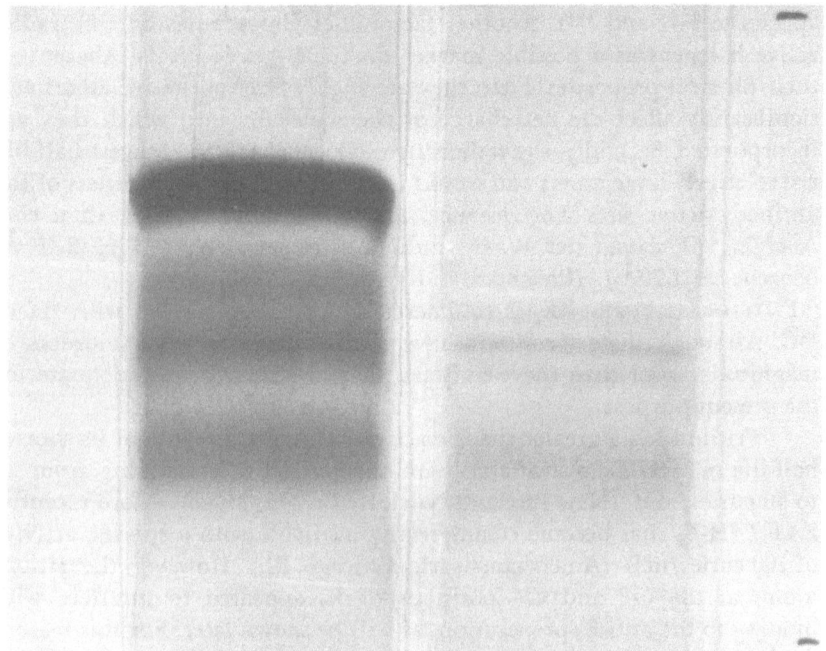

Fig. 2. Protein electrophoresis of S-41 anti-E_2 before and after Rivanol treatment.

Protein determinations were performed on the antiserum before and after Rivanol treatment, and were, respectively, 68 mg/ml and 25 mg/ml (corrected for dilution). This Rivanol-treated preparation contained 72 percent γ-globulins and 28 percent β-globulins. This treatment diluted the antiserum 1:5.

Antisera treated in this fashion were stable when kept frozen in 0.5 to 1 ml aliquots. After up to 2 years of storage at −20°C, no loss of binding activity has been detected. When needed, an aliquot was thawed, sodium azide added (at a concentration of 1 mg/ml) to prevent bacterial growth, and then stored at 4°C. After thawing, the antiserum was stable for up to 6 months when treated as described.

PREPARATION OF CELITE COLUMNS.   Celite (analytical filter aid, Johns Manville, Owens, Ill.) was prepared for use by heating at 1,000°F for at least 16 hours in an oven (Kushinsky and Paul, 1969). The celite was kept in the oven at this temperature until used. Disposable 5 ml graduated glass pipettes 5 mm in diameter (Kimble Glass Company, Owens, Ill.) were used only once. A small glass bead was used to block the lower end of the pipette which was then packed firmly to a height of 5 cm with a mixture of celite:ethylene glycol, 2:1 w/v in small (100 mg) aliquots, using isooctane as solvent. After packing, the columns were washed twice with 3.5 ml of isooctane prior to use for chromatography.

COUNTING FLUID AND COUNTING EQUIPMENT.   The liquid scintillation counting fluid used was prepared by mixing the following reagents in a large glass bottle:

> 300 ml of Biosolve BBS (Beckman, Fullertown, Calif.)
> 126 ml of Liquifluor (Pilot Chemical, Boston, Mass.)
> 3,000 ml of toluene (J. T. Baker, Phillipsburg, N.J.)

An automatic dilutor (Lab Industries, Berkeley, Calif.) was adapted to the neck of the bottle. When 10 ml of this preparation was used to solubilize 0.5 ml of assay buffer, an efficiency for ^{3}H-counting of 40 percent was obtained with a Packard liquid scintillation counter, Model 34322, with background of about 20 cpm. All samples were counted long enough to accumulate at least 2,500 cpm above background.

METHODS

Characterization of the Reagents

PREPARATION OF ANTIBODY-COATED TUBES.   Disposable polystyrene test tubes 10 by 75 mm (Falcon Plastics, Los Angeles, Calif.) were placed in the vertical position in a plastic rack designed to hold about 250 tubes

(Odell et al., 1967). The Rivanol-treated antiserum was then diluted with the coating buffer, the proper dilution being dictated by the titer curve. A volume of 0.4 ml of this diluted preparation was then added to the plastic test tubes in triplicate for each dilution. The tubes were incubated at 4°C for 16 hours. After incubation and careful removal of the coating solution by suction, 0.4 ml of the assay buffer was added and the tubes were placed at 4°C for 4 to 6 hours. The assay buffer was then aspirated and 0.6 ml of the same buffer added. Afterwards, these antibody-coated tubes could be stored at 4°C for up to 4 weeks prior to use. The rate of absorption of the antibodies to the tubes was found to be dependent upon the concentration of proteins used. Figure 3 shows the rate of coating when three different concentrations of protein were used. The same preparation used for coating was labeled with ^{125}I to a specific activity of 10 μc/μg by the method of Greenwood et al. (1963). A tracer amount of this preparation (5 ng) was added to each tube and the percent of tracer coated at different time intervals was evaluated. Since the protein concentration was known (25 mg/ml undiluted), the mass of protein coated at these time intervals could be calculated. It was found that the same mass of protein was coated when 1 and 10 μg (dilutions 1/10,000 and 1/1,000) were used, but that a lower mass was coated when 0.5 μg (dilution 1/20,000) was added. No matter how high the concentration of protein used, the mass coated never exceeded 650 ng. The

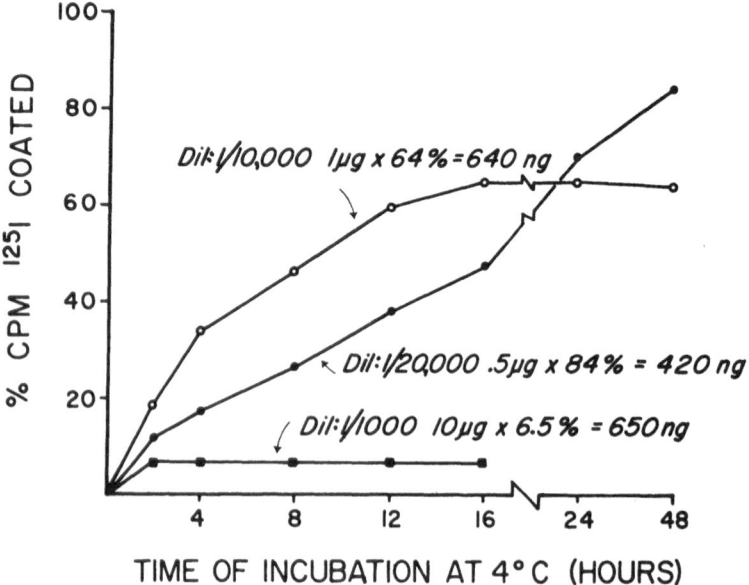

Fig. 3. Mass of proteins coated to plastic tubes when various dilutions of antiserum S-41 were used.

following calculations suggest that the mass of 650 ng represents the mass of γ-G (7S) (molecular weight=170,000) required to form a monolayer over the coated surface which was estimated to be about 2.3 cm². The following assumptions were made:

(1) The radioisotope ^{125}I was evenly distributed among antibodies and contaminant proteins in the Rivanol-treated preparation.

(2) The average molecular weight of the protein unit was 170,000.

(3) The size of γ-G (7S) represented the average size of the protein mixture—an ellipse with diameters 44 Å and 235 Å (Oncley et al., 1947).

(4) The protein molecules were absorbed over their largest surface: $235 \times 44 \times 10^{-16}$ cm² $\simeq 9.6 \times 10^{-13}$ cm² (rectangular surface).

With the above assumptions, the number of protein molecules required to form a monolayer over a surface of 2.3 cm² =

$$\frac{2.3 \text{ cm}^2}{9.6 \times 10^{-3} \text{ cm}^2} = 2.4 \times 10^{12} \text{ molecules,}$$

which represents

$$\frac{2.4 \times 10^{12} \text{ molecules}}{6.023 \times 10^{23} \text{ molecules/mole}} = 4 \times 10^{-12} \text{ mole,}$$

which has a mass of

$$\frac{170,000\text{g} \times 4}{\text{mole}} \times 10^{-12} \text{ mole} \times \frac{10^9 \text{ng}}{\text{g}} = 6.80 \times 10^2 \text{ ng.} = 680 \text{ ng.}$$

This value of 680 ng is surprisingly close to the value of 650 ng found experimentally, when one takes into consideration all the above assumptions, and is good evidence in favor of a monolayer system.

TESTING TITER.   Since the efficiency of the counter used for ^3H was about 40 percent, and the specific activity of the 6,7 ^3H-E_2 was 42 curies/ mM, a mass of 1 pg would give about 133 cpm. It was decided to use 5,000 cpm of 6,7 ^3H-E_2 (hereafter referred to as ^3H-E_2) in the assay. The mass of this tracer was about 40 pg. For testing the titer, various dilutions of the antibody preparation were used to coat the plastic tubes as described earlier. These coated tubes were then incubated at room temperature for 2 hours with 40 pg (5,000 cpm) of labeled tracer in 0.5 ml of assay buffer. The dilution that could bind 50 percent of this labeled tracer was used in the assay. A dilution of 1:20,000 was required to achieve this (Fig. 4). About 200 tubes were coated in one batch and the precision of coating for each batch was tested by an analysis of the percent cpm free after incubation of the labeled tracer without standard E_2 in 0.5 ml of assay buffer, using 10 replicate determinations. Tubes were used in the assay if the coefficient of variation was less than 5 percent.

EFFECT OF TEMPERATURE AND TIME OF INCUBATION ON BINDING OF ^3H-E_2 TO ANTI-E_2.   For this study, 40 pg of ^3H-E_2 was used as tracer and the

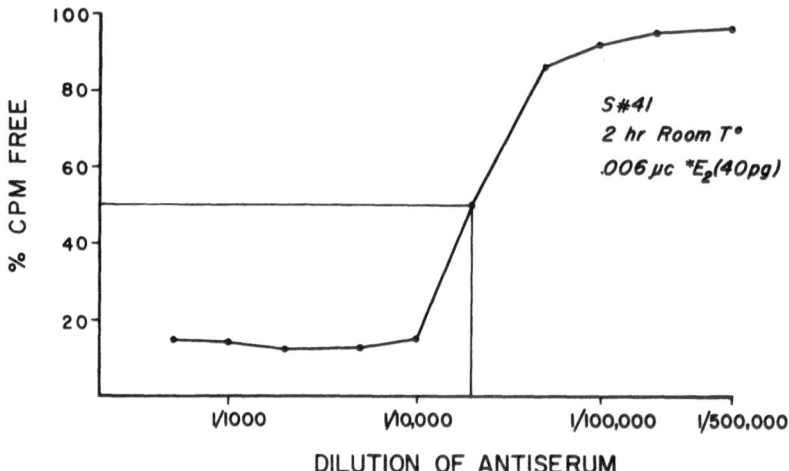

Fig. 4. Dose-response curve of dilution of antiserum used to coat tubes and the percent free E_2 when tubes were used for assay. A dilution of 1:20,000 was adequate to bind 50 percent of 40 pg ^{3}H-E_2.

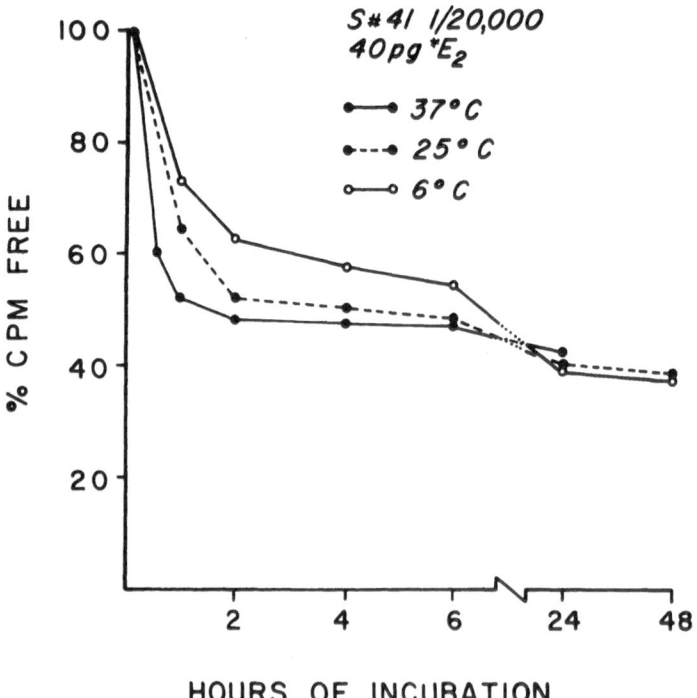

Fig. 5. Effect of temperature and time of incubation on binding of ^{3}H-E_2 to the antibody-coated tubes.

tubes were coated with a dilution of 1:20,000. Incubation was performed in 0.5 ml of assay buffer at three different temperatures (6°, 25°, and 37°C) for up to 48 hours. During the first few hours of incubation, the binding of ^{3}H-E_2 was greater at higher temperatures, but by 24 hours, the binding was about the same at all three temperatures (Fig. 5). No detectable increase in binding was noted after 24 hours of incubation. In order to insure that equilibrium had been achieved, the incubation was carried on for 24 hours in the thermodynamic studies. However, since the rate of change was minimal after 2 hours of incubation, except at 6°C, the incubation time for the assay was limited to 2 hours at room temperature.

EFFECT OF TIME OF INCUBATION AT ROOM TEMPERATURE ON THE SENSITIVITY OF THE ASSAY.   When E_2 was added in increasing amounts (from 2 to 400 pg) to antibody-coated tubes (dilution 1:20,000) and incubated in 0.5 ml of assay buffer at room temperature for 2 hours and 16 hours, it was found that the longer incubation time increased the sensitivity of the standard curve twofold (Fig. 6). However, as will be shown, the

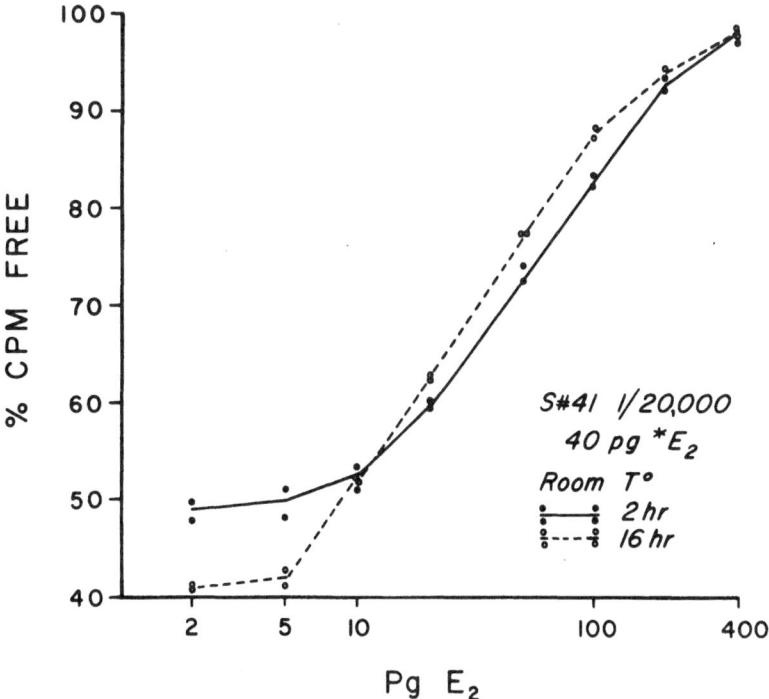

Fig. 6. Effect of incubation time on the sensitivity of radioimmunoassay of E_2.

limiting factor in the assay sensitivity of plasma samples was the level of the blank values, and the recovery of E_2 in these samples.

THERMODYNAMIC STUDIES.   The interaction of a low-molecular-weight hapten with an antibody-combining site may be expressed by the following equation: $H + B = HB$ in which H represents the hapten, B the antibody-combining site, and HB the antibody-bound hapten. The equilibrium constant for this reaction expressed as an association constant is:

$$K = \frac{[HB]}{[H][B]} \tag{1}$$

[ ] meaning molar concentration. At half-saturation of the antibody active sites, $HB = B$ and equation (1) becomes:

$$K = \frac{1}{H} \tag{2}$$

Antibody-coated tubes at a dilution of 1/20,000 coating solution were used for the thermodynamic studies.

When 6,7 ^{3}H-E_2 and 2,4,6,7 ^{3}H-E_2 were added in increasing amounts to 0.5 ml of assay buffer and incubated for 24 hours at 25°C in the antibody-coated tubes, 10 times less mass of free, 6,7 ^{3}H-E_2 than of 2,4,6,7-

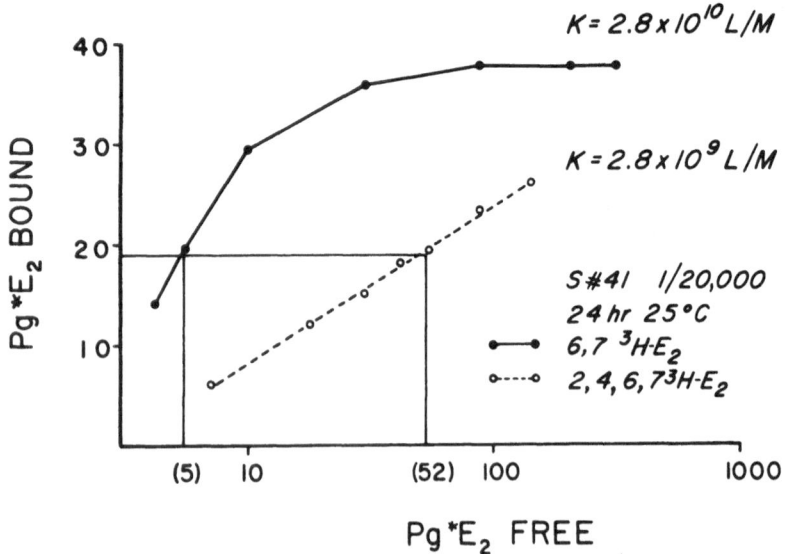

Fig. 7. Saturation experiments using two preparations of labeled E_2. (See text for further details.)
$^*E_2 = {}^3$H-E_2

^{3}H-E$_2$ was present at half-saturation of the antibody sites. Using equation (2) the K values for the two preparations of ^{3}H-E$_2$ were calculated (Fig. 7). They were, respectively: K = 2.8 × 10^{10} liter/M and 2.8 × 10^9 liter/M for 6,7 ^{3}H-E$_2$ and 2,4,6,7 ^{3}H-E$_2$.

Increasing amounts of E$_2$ and ^{3}H-E$_2$ were added to 40 pg ^{3}H-E$_2$ and incubated for 2 hours at room temperature. The percent cpm free was plotted against the logarithm of the mass added, and it was found that unlabeled E$_2$ was more effective in competitively displacing ^{3}H-E$_2$ than was ^{3}H-E$_2$ itself. The ^{3}H-E$_2$ displacement effect was 80 percent that of E$_2$ (Fig. 8). It is of interest to note that the small difference in size between hydrogen and tritium was sufficient to affect the binding of anti-E$_2$ to ^{3}H-E$_2$. However, this effect was much more pronounced when the tritium atoms were placed on ring A at the 2 and 4 positions than when placed on ring B at the positions 6, 7, suggesting a high tightness of fit between the anti-E$_2$ active site and ring A of E$_2$.

Since K for ^{3}H-E$_2$ = 2.8 × 10^{10} liter/M, the standard free energy ΔF^0 was calculated in the usual manner:

$$\Delta F^0 = -RT \ln k \qquad (3)$$

in which R is the gas constant and T the absolute temperature. When

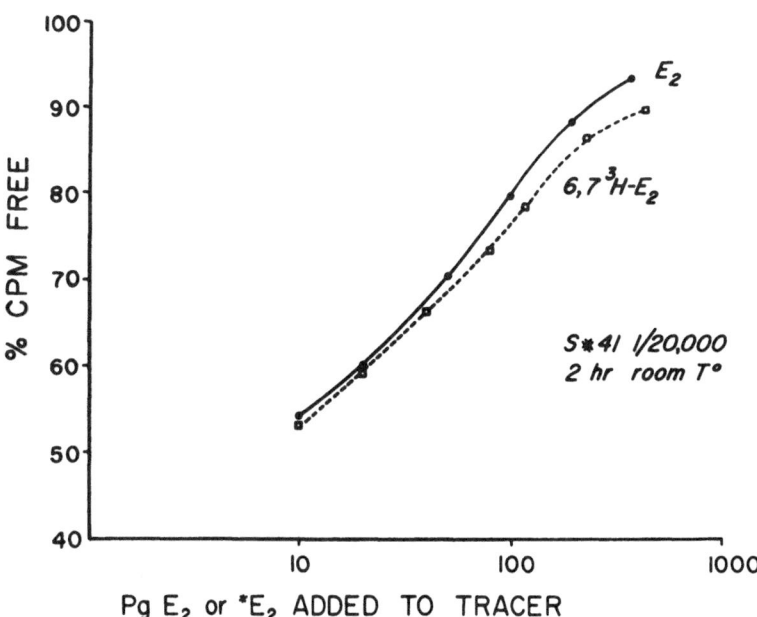

Fig. 8. Comparative effect of nonradioactive E$_2$ and tritiated *E$_2$ on the displacement of ^{3}H-E$_2$ from the antibody-coated tubes.

measurements of K at two temperatures are made, the enthalpy, ΔH^0, may be calculated using the integrated equation:

$$\log_{10} \frac{K_2}{K_1} = \frac{\Delta H^0}{2.303} \frac{(T_2 - T_1)}{RT_2 \cdot T_1} \tag{4}$$

and the entropy, ΔS^0, could be derived by the equation:

$$\Delta S^0 = \frac{\Delta H^0 - \Delta F^0}{T} \tag{5}$$

At 25°C, $K = 2.8 \times 10^{10}$ liter/M and at 6°C, $K = 3.4 \times 10^{10}$ liter/M.

Using equations (3), (4), and (5), the following values were obtained:

$\Delta F^0 = -14.2$ Kcal/mole

$\Delta H^0 = -1.6$ Kcal/mole

$\Delta S^0 = 42$ entropy units/mole.

Haptens with apolar groups such as benzene have been reported to give high positive entropy values (Karush, 1962). Such a high ΔS^0 could account for almost all the ΔF^0, and therefore this reaction is entropy driven. Assuming that the anti-E_2 has a molecular weight of 170,000, is divalent, and has both binding sites available for binding, the mass of anti-E_2 coated on the tubes could be calculated by saturating the sites with ^3H-E_2. When this experiment was performed (Table 3), the calcu-

TABLE 3

Comparative Study between the Mass of Proteins Coated to the Tubes and the Mass of ^3H-E_2-[a] Antibody Bound at Saturation

Dilution used for coating	Mass of proteins coated[b] in ng	Mass of ^3H-E_2[a] (pg) bound at saturation[c]	Calculated mass of anti-E_2 in ng[d]	Ratio of anti-E_2 coated to total protein coated
1/10,000	640	130	39	.06
1/15,000	420	85	25.5	.06
1/20,000	235	38	11.4	.05

[a] ^3H-E_2 = 6, 7, ^3H-Estradiol.

[b] Incubated 24 hours at 4°C for coating.

[c] Incubated 16 hours at room temperature for saturation experiments.

[d] Assuming that anti-E_2 has a M.W. = 170,000, is divalent, and both binding sites are available for binding.

lated mass of anti-E_2 coated was between 5 and 6 percent of the total protein coated. If our assumptions are correct, only 5 to 6 percent of the protein content of the Rivanol-treated preparation represents anti-E_2, giving a concentration of specific antibody of 25 mg $\times$ 5.5/100 = 1.37 mg/ml (undiluted antiserum).

Assay Procedure

EXTRACTION AND CHROMATOGRAPHIC PURIFICATION OF E_2.   Volumes of 0.1 to 5 ml of plasma or serum were used, depending on the expected level of E_2 in the plasma samples. Serum was preferred since it was easier to extract, had less emulsion and gel formations, and gave a higher recovery of E_2. However, no systematic study has been performed to compare values of E_2 obtained when plasma and serum samples from the same source are measured. When less than 2 ml of plasma was used, the volume was brought to 2 ml with water. A total of about 500 cpm of ^3H-E_2 in 0.1 ml of water was added to each sample and mixed. This ^3H-E_2 served as the internal standard for correction of recovery of E_2. Afterwards, extraction was carried out using three times 3 volumes of ether by mixing with a vortex mixer for 30 seconds. The pooled ether extract was evaporated to dryness under a stream of nitrogen and the residue redissolved in 0.2 to 0.5 ml of isooctane.

The isooctane was transferred to the celite column. The tubes were washed once more with 0.2 to 0.5 ml of isooctane and the latter transferred to the column. Elution was carried out under nitrogen pressure (6 to 8 drops/min) and the eluate discarded. Following this, 3.5 ml of isooctane were added and eluted. This fraction contained progesterone, Δ^5pregnenolone, and cholesterol. Elution with 3.5 ml of 15 percent ethylacetate in isooctane removed estrone, 17-hydroxyprogesterone, 20α-hydroxy-4-pregnene-3-one, testosterone, androstenedione, and 5α-dihydrotestosterone. Three and one-half milliliters of 40 percent ethylacetate in isooctane eluted E_2 and estradiol-17α. Among the steroids tested, estradiol-17α was found to be the only contaminant of the E_2 fraction. Estriol remained on the column, and could be eluted with 3.5 ml of ethylacetate.

DETECTION OF E_2.   The dried extract of the E_2 fraction was dissolved in 1 ml of assay buffer and 0.4 ml was added to a counting vial containing 0.1 ml of assay buffer. This served as the internal standard and represented 40 percent of the E_2 present in the extract. Another 0.4 ml aliquot was added to the antibody-coated tubes, and 0.1 ml of ^3H-E_2 (5,000 cpm) in assay buffer was added and mixed. Incubation was carried out at room temperature for 2 hours. Afterwards, the incubation medium was quantitatively transferred to a counting vial and diluted in 10 ml of counting fluid, using an automatic dilutor. All samples were counted long enough to have a counting error of less than 2 percent. Four water samples, run together with the plasma samples, served as a check on the blank of the method. All samples were measured by interpolation on a standard curve, run together with the unknown samples and the blanks. Blank values of 20 pg E_2 or less were considered as acceptable in the assay. If the blanks were over 20 pg E_2, a systematic check on the solvents and celite was carried out. In our experience, the only source of significantly high blanks has been the ethylacetate.

RESULTS

Reliability Experiments

SPECIFICITY.   Specificity of an assay system refers to its ability to respond only to the hormone which the assay is intended to quantify. Absolute specificity is difficult to demonstrate. If a partially nonspecific detection system is used, adequate specificity can be expected if the purification steps performed prior to detection remove all the known contaminants that interfere. We have previously presented data (Abraham, 1969) concerning the specificity of the antiserum. It reacted only with estradiol-17β, estradiol-17α, estrone, and estriol. Nonestrogenic steroids and the nonsteroid estrogen, diethylstilbestrol, failed to react significantly. Although estrogen conjugates are possible sources of interference, they were removed by the ether extraction; estrogen conjugates are not extracted from aqueous solutions and plasma using this solvent (Preedy, 1968) . The two cross-reacting estrogens, estrone and estriol, are separated from E_2 by the chromatographic step. The only known contaminant in the E_2 fraction is estradiol-17α, which showed a 35 percent cross-reaction with the antiserum used. However, to our knowledge, free estradiol-17α has not been isolated from human blood. In species known to have this estrogen in the free form in their biologic fluids, this assay would not be specific for E_2.

It is possible that some synthetic estrogens might interfere with this assay, and care must be exercised when measuring E_2 in patients on these medications. Diethylstilbestrol cross-reacted less than .01 percent with this antiserum, but 17α-ethinyl-estradiol-17β cross-reacted 6 percent and is not separated from E_2 by the chromatographic system used. Therefore, at least one of the synthetic estrogens is a possible interfering material if the blood level of this compound is high enough.

Comparative measurements of E_2 made on the same plasma samples, using this method and a double-isotope assay (Baird, 1968) showed no systematic difference between the two assays (Table 4) . When E_2 was measured in plasma samples obtained from women on high-dose progestin medication, the values obtained compared favorably with those obtained by another competitive protein-binding assay, using rabbit uterine cytosol as specific-binding protein (Korenman et al., 1969) .

SENSITIVITY.   Although 10 pg E_2 was significantly different from 0 pg E_2 on the standard curve, the sensitivity of the assay in the measurement of E_2 in unknown samples was dependent on both the blank values and

TABLE 4

Comparison of the Double-Isotope Method
with the Radioimmunoassay of Estradiol-17-β

Sample number	Double-isotope assay[a] (pg/ml plasma)	Radioimmunoassay (pg/ml plasma)
1	24.5	<25
2	33.9	<25
3	461	425
4	4157	>3850
5	619	685
6[b]	118	136
7	1065	1220
8	2001	1945
9	6410	>3580

[a]Performed by the method of Baird, 1968. J. Clin. Endocr., 28:244-258. Samples kindly supplied by Dr. C.W. Lloyd and Miss J. Lobotsky, who did the measurement of E_2 by the double-isotype method.

[b]All samples except No. 6 are from human ovarian veins. Sample No. 6 is peripheral venous plasma.

the recovery of E_2. If the blanks were less than the sensitivity of the standard curve (about 10 pg E_2) they were not subtracted from the unknown samples. However, since the blanks could have any value from 0 to 10 pg of E_2, it was recognized that overestimation of E_2 was a possibility. This was particularly true in those cases where the measurements made were at the level of assay sensitivity. When the blank values were measurable (between 10 and 20 pg of E_2), the mean ± S.D. of the four replicate samples was calculated. This mean value of the blank was subtracted from that of unknown samples prior to correction for recovery, and the sensitivity was then considered to be equal to two S.D. of the mean of the blank, and was usually between 6 and 10 pg of E_2. Since only 40 percent of the E_2 fraction was used in the assay, the recovery ranged from 22 to 34 percent. The recovery was significantly higher when serum samples were used [31.5 ± 1.3 (S.E.) for six serum samples, compared with 25.6±2.3 (S.E.) for six plasma samples].

After correction for recovery, the sensitivity per sample measured varied between 25 and 50 pg of E_2. When increasing amounts of E_2 were added to 2 ml of pooled male plasma and measured in the assay (Fig. 9), the smallest amount of E_2 that could consistently be recovered quantitatively was 50 pg. Therefore, for all practical purposes, the sensitivity of the assay was 50 pg, although as little as 25 pg E_2/sample could sometimes be measured.

PRECISION.   Plasma samples from different sources were measured for E_2, using samples volumes of 1 to 5 ml. When either 1 or 2 ml of pooled plasma from eugonadal men was used, the level of E_2 was undetectable (Table 5). With a volume of 5 ml, however, the amount of E_2 measured was 18 ± 2.4 (S.D.) pg/ml, giving a coefficient of variation of 13 percent (quadruplicate determinations).

Using pooled plasma from eugonadal women (follicular phase), 1 ml of serum was sufficient to measure E_2; a mean of 74 ± 8.6 pg/ml was obtained. The coefficient of variation was 12 percent. When larger volumes of plasma were measured, the precision improved, giving coefficients of variation as low as 4 percent.

ACCURACY.   The accuracy of the assay was tested by the recovery of E_2 added to plasma from men (Fig. 9). Regression analysis of the data gave the curve y = 0.92x + 26. The intercept of the line with the y axis gave a value of 26 pg of E_2, corresponding approximately to the level of E_2 present in 2 ml of the plasma used.

Practicability of the Assay

The practicability of an assay is judged by the skill required to perform it, the time involved in its use, and the cost of the assay. Although no special skill is required for this assay, meticulous attention to cleanli-

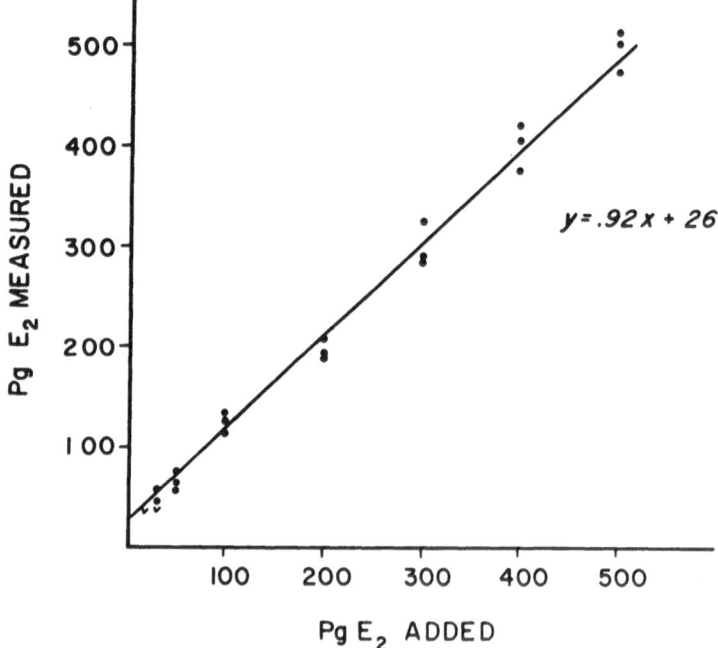

Fig. 9.   Recovery of known amounts of E_2 added to 2 ml of male plasma as measured in the assay. The equation y = 0.92x + 26 was obtained by regression analysis.

TABLE 5

Precision Experiments

Source of plasma samples	Volume of plasma used	[a]pg E_2/ml plasma ± S.D.
I. Pool male	1 ml	$<45, <30, <45, <45$
	2 ml	$<25, <22, 24, <20$
	5 ml	18 ± 2.4
II. Pool female	1 ml	74 ± 8.6
(follicular)	2 ml	68 ± 4.1
	5 ml	63 ± 2.8
III. Pool female	1 ml	192 ± 14
(luteal)	2 ml	178 ± 8.5

[a]All samples run in quadruplicate.

ness, awareness of the possible sources of interference, and consistency in the performance of this assay are qualities which an assayist must have. In an 8-hour working day, one person can run the assay on 24 samples, including four water blanks. A manifold was designed to hold 24 columns of celite (Fig. 10) and the same manifold served as a drying apparatus. The cost per sample was estimated to be between 65 and 80

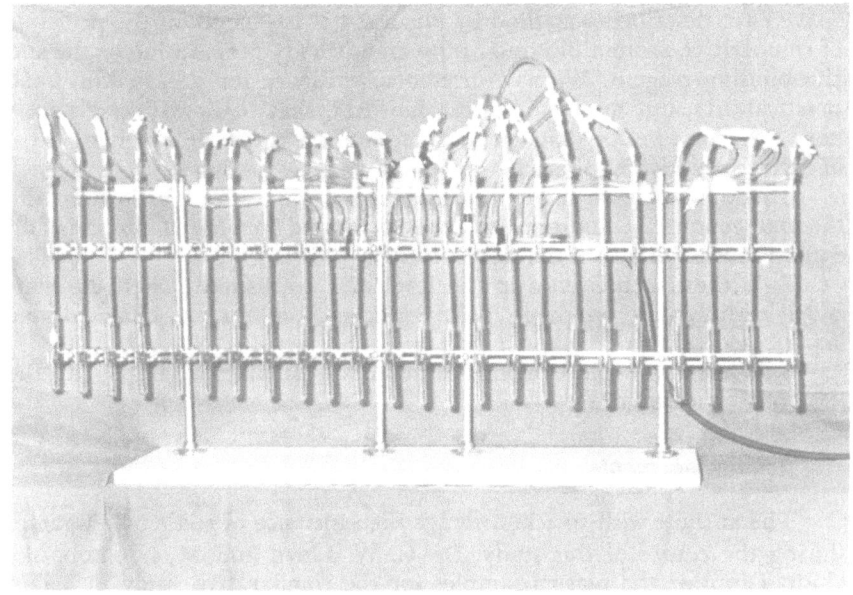

Fig. 10. Manifold designed to hold 24 columns of celite. The same equipment placed in a hood may be used as a drying apparatus. Nitrogen under pressure is used to accelerate elution.

cents, assuming a rate of 60 unknown samples a week, and excluding the cost of the liquid scintillation counter, which was the most expensive item used in the assay.

DISCUSSION

One of the greatest needs in the field of endocrinology is the improvement of methodology to increase sensitivity of hormone measurement without loss of reliability. Especially for clinical investigations, the volume of blood required for an assay should be less than 10 ml, and the sensitivity of the assay dictates the volume of the sample. Another important aspect is the practicability of an assay since the widespread acceptance of an assay depends on this criterion. The more recent detection methods, using specific-binding proteins as reagents (Berson and Yalow, 1959; Ekins, 1960; Murphy, 1964; Korenman et al., 1969; Abraham, 1969), seem to fulfill the requirements for reliability and practicability. Among the specific proteins used, immunoglobulins are the most stable, the best characterized, and therefore seem to be the best suited for this type of assay. They have been proven to be a powerful tool when applied to the measurement of polypeptide hormones. All hormones are probably immunogenic under some circumstances and thus this approach can be used to quantify all hormones.

We have described a method for the assay of E_2, based on the principle of competitive-protein binding, using an antibody preparation as the specific-binding reagent. We have presented evidence for its reliability and practicability, but must emphasize, however, that this assay is relatively new. It has not been exhaustively tested and we conclude by giving a list of some aspects which should be investigated:

1. Is the labeled E_2 added to the plasma samples in equilibrium with the endogenous E_2, and are they equally bound to plasma proteins and equally extractable with the solvents used?

2. Is there a difference in the level of E_2 measured, when the same blood samples are prepared differently, such as serum, oxalated and heparinized plasma?

3. What is the effect of long-term storage of plasma samples on the level of E_2 measured?

Acknowledgments

The authors wish to acknowledge the assistance of some investigators during the course of this study. Dr. C. W. Lloyd and Miss J. Lobotsky kindly supplied the plasma samples for the comparative study in Table 4. We appreciate the use of the liquid scintillation counter and numerous helpful suggestions made by Dr. S. G. Korenman. The thermodynamic studies were performed with the expert assistance of Dr. R. M. Nakamura, who also enriched our study by numerous pleasant discussions and suggestions. We thank Mrs. D. Fisher for her expert preparation of the manuscript.

REFERENCES

Abraham, G. E. 1969. Solid-phase radioimmunossay of estradiol-17β. J. Clin. Endocr., 29:866–870.

Baird, D. T. 1968. A method for the measurement of estrone and estradiol-17β in peripheral human blood and other biological fluids using ^{35}S-pipsylchloride. J. Clin. Endocr., 28:244–258.

Berson, S. A., and R. S. Yalow. 1959. Assay of plasma insulin in human subjects by immunological methods. Nature (London), 184:1648.

Ekins, R. P. 1960. The estimation of thyroxine in human plasma by an electrophoretic technique. Clin. Chim. Acta, 5:453.

Greenwood, F. C., W. M. Hunter, and J. S. Glover. 1963. The preparation of ^{131}I-labelled human growth hormone of high specific radioactivity. Biochem. J., 89:114.

Karush, F. 1962. Immunologic specificity and molecular structure. *In* Taliaferro, W. H., and J. H. Humphrey, eds. Advances in Immunology, Vol. 2, 1–39, New York, Academic Press, Inc.

Korenman, S. G., L. E. Perrin, and T. P. McCullum. 1969. A radioligand binding assay system for estradiol measurement in human plasma. J. Clin. Endocr., 29:879–883.

Kushinsky, S., and W. Paul. 1969. Use of a "self-cleaning" oven to clean liquid scintillation vials and other glassware. Anal. Biochem., 30:465–467.

Murphy, B. E. P. 1964. The application of the property of protein-binding to the assay of minute quantities of hormones and other substances. Nature (London), 201:679.

Odell, W. D., P. L. Rayford, and G. T. Ross. 1967. Simplified partially automated method for radioimmunoassay of human TSH, GH, LH, and FSH. J. Clin. Med., 70:973–980.

Oncley, J. L., G. Scatchard, and A. Brown. 1947. Physicochemical characteristics of certain of the proteins of normal human plasma. J. Phys. Colloid Chem., 51:184–198.

Preedy, J. R. K. 1968. Estrogens. *In* Dorfman, R. I., ed. Methods in Hormone Research, 2nd ed. 1–64, New York, Academic Press, Inc.

Pressman, D., and A. Grossberg. 1968. The Structural Basis of Antibody Specificity. New York, W. A. Benjamin, Inc.

DISCUSSION

K. CATT.   We have no experience with the immunoassay of steroids but there are some examples obtained in our work on protein hormones which are very consistent with the results Dr. Abraham has presented.

In terms of the nature of the antibody coating, we also looked some time ago at the relationship between the antibody mass attached to the tube and the ability of the coated tubes to bind labeled tracer, in this case human growth hormone. When the antibody was trace labeled with ^{125}I rabbit gamma globulin and used to coat tubes in various concentrations the family of curves was obtained shown in Figure 1. These curves were derived by plotting the duration of coating against the antibody mass which can be calculated to be attached to the tube. You can see that the more concentrated solutions, as would be expected, coat more rapidly and more heavily.

If these antibody-coated tubes are then incubated with ^{131}I-human-growth-hormone tracer, we can show that the rate of attachment of labeled antigen is relatively more rapid than that of the labeled antibody. Thus, there is a difference between the rate of adsorption of

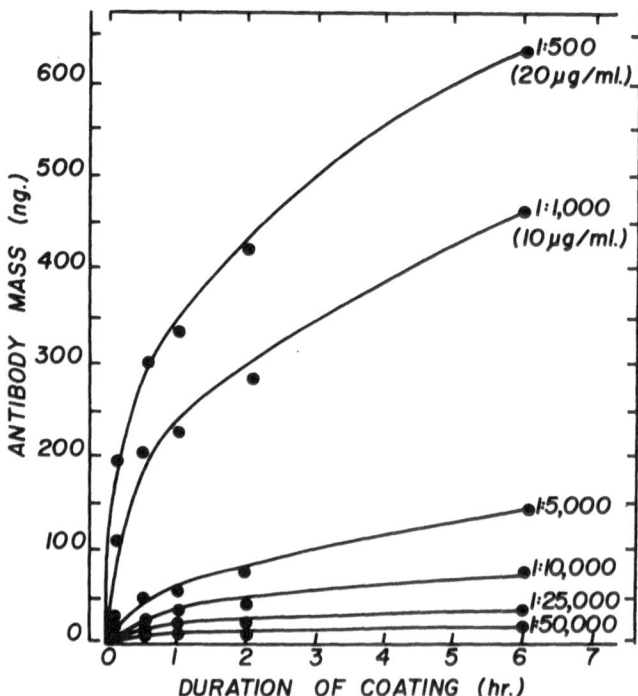

Fig. 1.   Binding of antibodies to plastic tubes after various dilutions of the antisera.

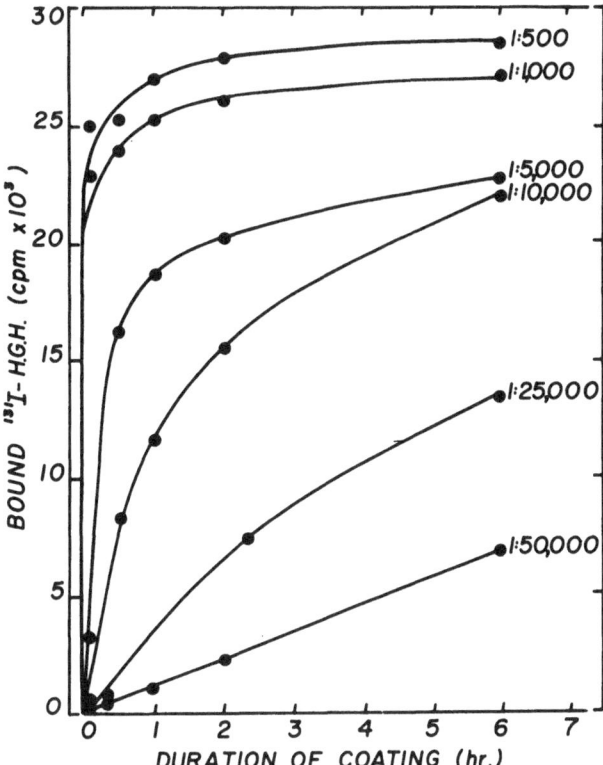

Fig. 2. Binding of HGH (human growth hormone) to HCG antibodies coated to plastic tubes.

antibody and the ability of this antibody to combine with tracer (Fig. 2).

If we construct from these families of curves a relationship between the mass of bound antigen and the antibody adsorbed to the tube, it is apparent that beyond a certain level of antibody adsorption, in this case about 100 ng, there is no further increase in antigen binding. This could be caused by steric hindrance in the presence of densely packed antibody molecules, or by adsorption occurring in a layered fashion with only the surface layer available for reaction with antigen (Fig. 3).

One or two other points about Dr. Abraham's results: With regard to the irreversibility of the system, we observed in 1966 that once growth-hormone tracer was combined with solid-phase antibody, the addition of relatively enormous quantities of antigen, up to a million-fold excess, would not displace the labeled antigen from the solid-phase antibody. Thus, it seems that the solid-phase immune reactions are relatively much less reversible than the reaction in solution. This is most probably due to a reduced rate of dissociation as suggested by Dr. Abraham's results. I think that this relative irreversibility is one important reason why the

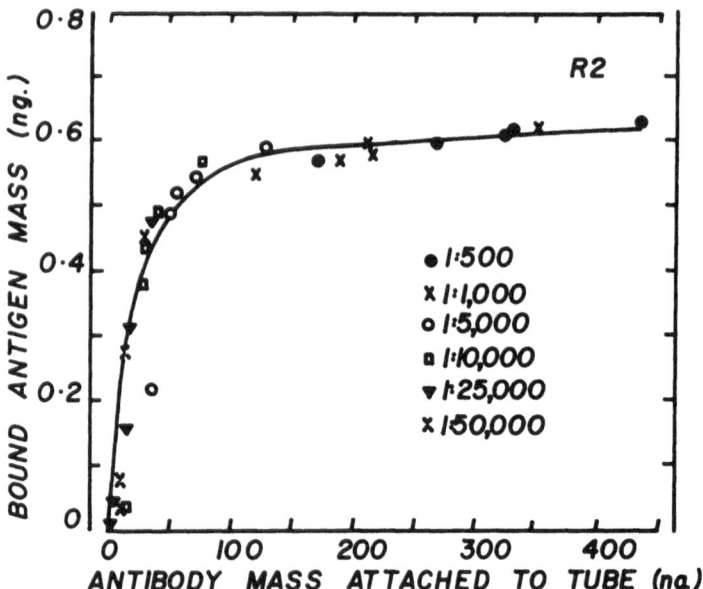

Fig. 3. Ratio of mass of bound antigen (HGH) to mass of antibody attached to tube at various dilutions.

solid-phase systems function so well despite the less intimate contact between antigen in solution and antibody attached to the tube surface, compared to the situation when both are in solution.

Finally, for counting such solid-phase systems, it is possible to coat plastic beta-counting vials with antibody, perform assays in such vials, then simply wash out the vial and add an appropriate scintillator to obtain the bound count. On the other hand, to count the free hormone it is possible to partition estradiol or testosterone rapidly into the standard toluene scintillator and count directly.

G. ABRAHAM.   We did not have to extract out of the aqueous medium with toluene because we use Biosolve which solubilizes this aqueous material in toluene. Some people have used a two-phase counting system in toluene.

S. GROSS.   I am almost beginning to believe in radioimmunoassay after Dr. Abraham's presentation. However, there are a few points I would like to have clarified. Your calculations, if I understood correctly, depended upon the fact that your tyrosine had been known to iodinate equally on your immunoglobulin and on your monolayers. Is that right?

G. ABRAHAM.   The specific activity, as you recall, was only 10 μc μg. Assuming that the isotope abundance that the suppliers gave us is true, the ratio was 0.2 atom of iodine per mole of IgG and under these conditions, from the work of Pressman and others, the iodination did not affect significantly the characteristics of this protein.

S. GROSS.   I would think that the counts for the number of iodine atoms that are available per mole of IgG per mole would vary considerably. Some might have 20 residues of iodine, others may have one; and if that is true, then the arithmetic would have to be explained.

G. ABRAHAM.   We do not know that this iodination follows the Gaussian curve. When we say we have 0.2 atoms of iodine per molecule, obviously we cannot incorporate 0.2 atom. Therefore, the figure represents an average incorporation. Some protein molecules might have two, others none at all.

S. GROSS.   Moles of protein present per disc may not be a true Gaussian distribution.

G. ABRAHAM.   I realize that we had to make a lot of assumptions and we are pleased to see the values obtained experimentally correlated with the calculated one. In fact, we were even surprised.

E. KNOBIL.   Dr. Abraham, I wonder if you have had the opportunity to systematically compare recovery from plasma samples of tritiated versus cold estradiol. The reason I ask this question is that we found a much larger variation in recoveries with tritiated estradiol than cold estradiol and have come to the conclusion that, in our hands at least, the tritiated recoveries are quite unreliable. We suspect the reason for this is that, in most of the tritiated estradiol preparations that we have used, many of the counts recovered are not in the form of estradiol.

G. ABRAHAM.   When the tritium atoms are on ring A, I think they are very unstable. The 6,7^{3}H-estradiol seems to be much more stable.

M. LIPSETT.   Have you compared results with your system to those of Korenman's uterine cytosol-binding system? Do you get essentially the same results? Do you care to comment on the practicability of the two methods? What advantages does your method have over Korenman's?

G. ABRAHAM.   Well, as I mentioned, gamma globulin is more stable than uterine cytosol, and one can get a much greater affinity with antibodies. I believe, however, that each laboratory must make the decision as to which method is most reliable in their hands.

H. BRODIE.   With regard to Dr. Abraham's findings concerning the variable binding of estradiol tritiated at different positions, we have data supporting this conclusion. We found that incubation of 19-norandrostenedione-7β-^{3}H-4-^{14}C with a microorganism gave us some hydroxylated and keto steroids with tritium-^{14}C ratios much higher than the ratio in the starting material. The reason for this may be that the tritiated material is binding to an enzyme site better than the untritiated or the ^{14}C material, thus leading to faster conversion. It is worth noting also that Mahler, working with alcohol dehydrogenase, found that deuterated ethanol binds better to the enzyme than undeuterated material. This appears to be a real phenomenon worth keeping in mind in this work.

J. FISHMAN.   We have also observed the effect of tritium located at C-2 and C-4 on the binding of estradiol to proteins. In the case studied, location of tritium at C-2 or C-4, but not at C-16α, increased binding significantly when compared to estradiol-6,7 ^{3}H. The isotope effect need not be steric in origin; it is possible that it is due to electronic effects of the isotope transmitted by resonance to the phenolic group, altering its chemistry and particularly its acidity.

6

RADIOIMMUNOASSAY OF PLASMA ESTROGENS: USE OF POLYMERIZED ANTIBODIES

George Mikhail, Hsiu-Wu Chung

Department of Obstetrics and Gynecology
The University of Texas
Southwestern Medical School at Dallas
Dallas, Texas

Michel Ferin,* Raymond L. Vande Wiele

Department of Obstetrics and Gynecology
Columbia University College of Physicians and Surgeons
New York, New York

INTRODUCTION

Antibodies to estradiol can be produced by immunization of sheep with estradiol-17β-succinyl-bovine serum albumin (Ferin et al., 1968). The biologic potency of these antibodies in neutralizing circulating estrogens has been demonstrated by Ferin et al. (1968, 1969). The availability of steroid antibodies opened the possibility of their use in the development of radioimmunoassay of steroids. Preliminary results of radioimmunoassays of estradiol (Abraham, 1969) and testosterone (Niswender and Midgley, 1969) have been reported recently.

This work was supported in part by grants AM 11057 and HD 02996 from the National Institutes of Health.
* The International Institute for the Study of Human Reproduction.

An important step in any radioimmunoassay is the separation of free from protein-bound fractions. Several methods have been described for this purpose, including those using double antibodies (Bidgley et al., 1969), dry coating of plastic tubes with antiserum (Catt and Tregear, 1967), and polymerized antibodies. The last method has been employed by Donini et al. (1968) in radioimmunoassay of human chorionic gonadotropin. Though water-insoluble, polymerized protein antibodies were found to be efficient and stable immunoadsorbents (Avrameas and Ternynck, 1967).

This chapter deals with the development of a radioimmunoassay for plasma estrone and estradiol which is sensitive, specific, simple, and rapid. By means of this method, daily concentrations of plasma estrone and estradiol during the human menstrual cycle were determined.

PREPARATION OF ESTRONE AND ESTRADIOL ANTIBODY REAGENTS

The sera obtained from immunized sheep were initially absorbed with bovine serum albumin and then treated with Rivanol as recommended by Abraham (1969). The excess Rivanol was adsorbed with charcoal and the charcoal was removed by centrifugation. The treated antiserum was polymerized in the following manner: About 10 ml of the antiserum was transferred into a small beaker and 0.2 ml of ethyl chloroformate was added dropwise while the solution was stirred constantly. The reaction was monitored with a pH meter and 1 N NaOH was intermittently added to neutralize the acidifying effect of ethyl chloroformate. In about 30 minutes the solution became markedly turbid. The stability of the pH of the solution indicated the completion of the reaction. The polymerized antiserum was centrifuged at 10,000 rpm for 10 minutes and the supernatant was discarded. Exhaustive washing of the antibodies was carried out using 0.1 M phosphate buffer pH 7.2, 0.1 percent sodium carbonate, and 0.2 M glycine-HCl buffer pH 2.2 until the optical density of the washes at 280 mμ was less than 0.01. Final washes with phosphate buffer pH 7.2 brought the pH of the antiserum solution to neutrality. The purpose of these washes was to remove the excess ethyl chloroformate and to eliminate any soluble proteins which may interfere in the assay. The polymerized antiserum was then homogenized in a Teflon homogenizer. The homogenized suspension was diluted with phosphate buffer pH 7.2 to 10 times the original antiserum volume and was stored at 4°C for extended periods of time (over 6 months) without loss of

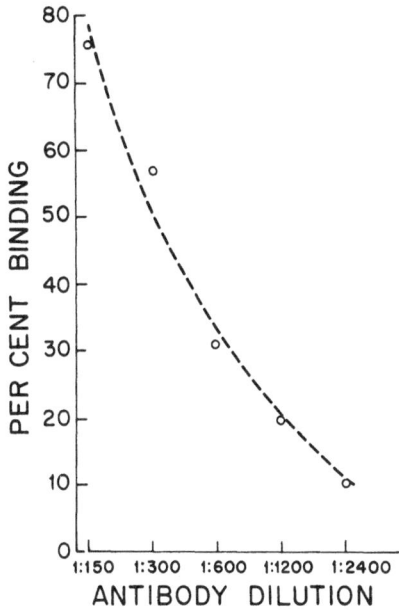

Fig. 1. Effect of the antibody titer on binding of ³H-estradiol.

potency. To test the titer of the antibodies, serial dilutions were made and their ability to bind ³H-estradiol was determined (Fig. 1). There was a progressive decrease in the binding capacity with increasing dilution of the antiserum.

The dilute antibody reagent that was used for the assay was prepared as follows: ³H-estradiol was dissolved in 100 ml of phosphate buffer pH 7.2 to a final concentration of 10,000 to 15,000 cpm/ml buffer. A suitable amount of estradiol antiserum of known titer was added and the mixture was shaken thoroughly and stored at 4°C. The stability of this antibody reagent was tested over a 4-month period, and satisfactory standard curves were obtained (Fig. 2) with minimal loss of binding capacity after 4 months of storage.

Early in our study it was found that estrone cross-reacted effectively with these estradiol antibodies. An estrone reagent was made by mixing ³H-estrone with estradiol antiserum and was used in conjunction with the estradiol reagent for the development of radioimmunoassay for both estrone and estradiol. Typical standard curves for estrone and estradiol obtained with the two reagents are shown in Figure 3.

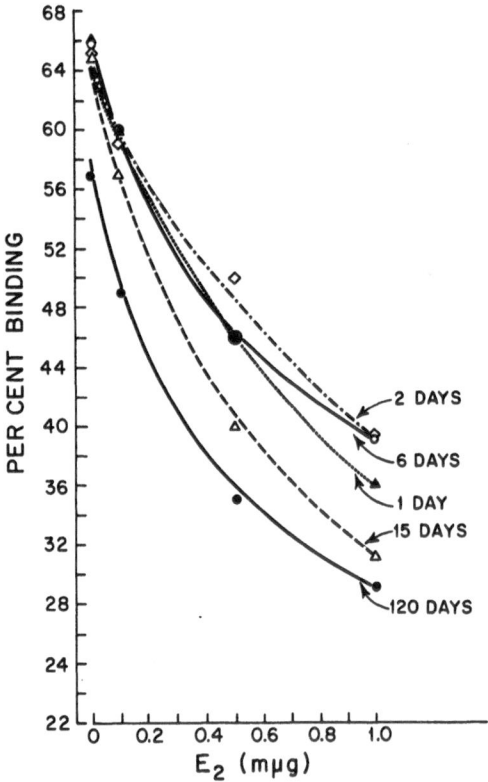

Fig. 2. Estradiol standard curves obtained in a period of 4 months using the same estradiol reagent. Figs. 2–8 from Mikhail. 1970. *Steroids*, 14:333–352. (Courtesy of Holden-Day, Inc.)

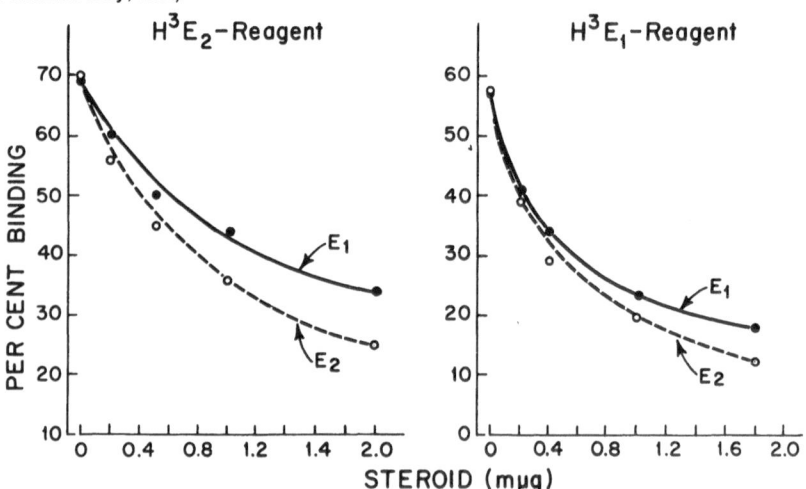

Fig. 3. Estrone and estradiol standard curves obtained with both the estrone and estradiol reagents.

EXTRACTION AND PURIFICATION OF PLASMA ESTROGENS

Purified ^{3}H-estradiol and/or ^{3}H-estrone were pipetted into extraction tubes and evaporated to dryness. Plasma (2 to 5 ml) was added and mixed with the tracer. After addition of carbonate buffer pH 9.5 (15 percent of volume), the mixture was extracted three times with an equal volume of fresh ether. The combined ether extract was washed twice with a 10 percent volume of water and evaporated to dryness. Column chromatography using Sephadex LH-20 was used for the separation of estrone and estradiol. Three grams of Sephadex LH-20 were suspended in a mixture of benzene:methanol (85:15) and transferred to a glass column (300 by 10 mm). The Sephadex column was initially washed with 300 to 400 ml of benzene:methanol to eliminate impurities which interfered with the assay. The columns were used repeatedly for a period of 3 to 6 months. Each volumn was eluted with 20 to 30 ml of solvent between sample applications. The elution pattern of a mixture of steroid tracers in a typical column is shown in Figure 4. Plasma extracts were transferred to the column with multiple small aliquots of benzene: methanol (85:15), eluted with the same solvent, and the estrone and/or estradiol fractions were collected. Aliquots of the column effluent equal

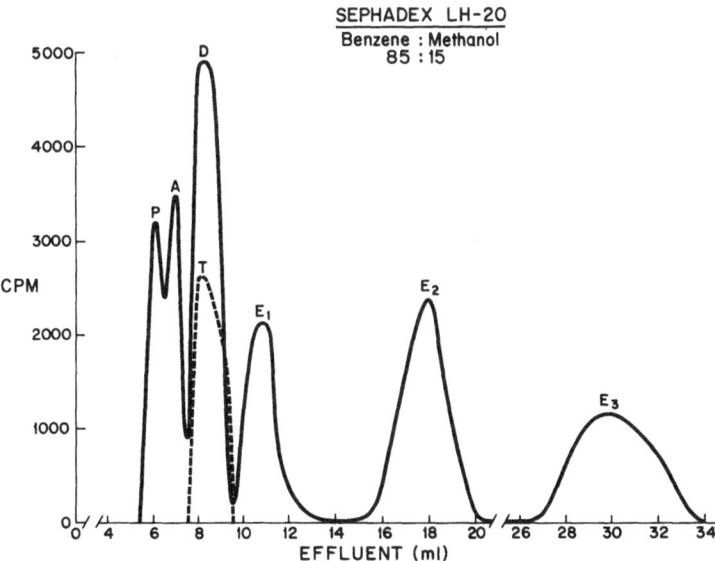

Fig. 4. Chromatographic behavior of steroid tracers in Sephadex LH-20 column. P=progesterone; A=androstenedione; D=dehydroepiandrosterone; T=testosterone; E_1=estrone; E_2=estradiol; and E_3=estriol.

in volume to the steroid fraction were initially collected prior to addition of the plasma extracts and were used as column elution blanks. The samples and the elution blanks were evaporated to dryness and dissolved in 0.7 ml of benzene: methanol; 0.15-ml aliquots were taken for measuring recovery of the added tracer and 0.5-ml aliquots were transferred to 3.5-ml polypropylene centrifuge tubes for the assay. Similarly, 0.5-ml aliquots of the elution blanks were added to tubes containing known amounts of estrone or estradiol which were used to construct the reference standard curve.

ASSAY PROCEDURE

The tubes containing the estrogen standards and unknown extracts were kept in an ice bath and 1 ml of the antibody reagent was added to each tube. It should be pointed out that the reagent is a suspension and not a solution; therefore, in order to insure the homogeneity of the suspension, the flask containing the reagent was thoroughly shaken prior to each pipetting. The efficiency of this step was tested by counting reagent aliquots obtained at the time of the first and last pipetting. These aliquots, representing the concentration of the tracer in the reagent, were also used to calculate the degree of binding. Incubation was carried out at room temperature for 2 hours and followed by centrifugation at 2 to 4°C for 10 minutes at 15,000 rpm. The tubes were returned to an ice

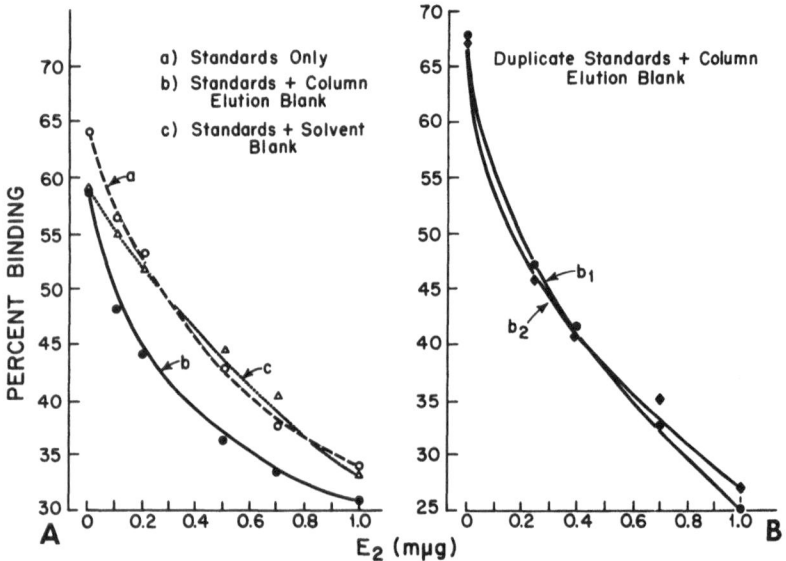

Fig. 5A and 5B. Effect of solvents and column elution blanks on standard curves.

bath and 0.4 ml of the supernatant, representing the free fraction, was pipetted into counting vials, mixed with 10 ml of a modified Bray's solution (Neill et al., 1967), and counted for 20 minutes. The standard curves were plotted as cpm free steroid or percent bound versus mµg of estradiol or estrone and used for determination of the unknown concentration of the steroid in the plasma samples. Results were corrected for experimental losses and the final concentration was expressed as picograms of estradiol or estrone per milliliter of plasma.

When aliquots of organic solvents (benzene, methanol) or column elution blanks were added to estradiol standards, the standard curves shown in Figure 5a were obtained. However, when column elution blanks collected from different Sephadex LH-20 columns were added to duplicate sets of estradiol standards, superimposable curves resulted (Fig. 5b). In view of these results, addition of column elution blanks to tubes containing the estrogen standards became an integral step in the assay.

RESULTS

The mean water blank was 14 ± 2 pg for estrone and 11 ± 1 pg for estradiol. Plasma from oophorectomized-adrenalectomized individuals was not available, therefore the plasma blank could not be estimated. However, in some postmenopausal plasma samples, we obtained estradiol values of less than 15 pg.

The lower limit of sensitivity of the method is approximately 50 pg. With recoveries ranging from 70 to 90 percent, it was possible to measure estrone and estradiol in 1 to 3 ml of female plasma.

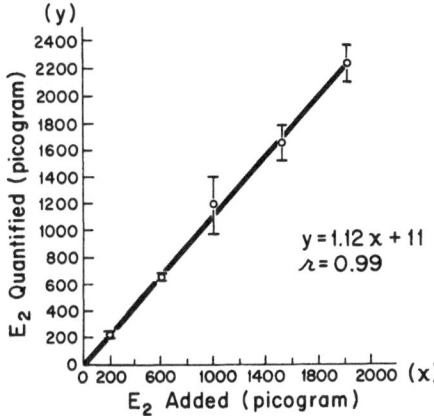

Fig. 6. Correlation between estradiol added to water and estradiol quantified. Each point represents the mean ± S.D. (Refer to Table 1.)

To test the accuracy and precision of the method, known amounts of estrone and estradiol were added to water and processed in a manner similar to that used for plasma, including extraction, column chromatography, and radioimmunoassay. A linear relationship was obtained between the estrone added and the estrone quantified: $Y = 1.02X + 14$. Similar results were obtained with estradiol (Fig. 6). In addition, replicate determinations of estrone and estradiol in plasma samples were

TABLE 1

Accuracy and Reproducibility of the Estradiol Method

	No. of determinations	Mean pg	Standard deviation	Standard error	Coefficient of variation (percent)
Water blank	7	11	1	0.4	9
Water + added estradiol					
100 pg	3	112	16	9.3	14
200 pg	7	231	20	7.5	9
600 pg	4	665	25	13.0	4
1000 pg	14	1,210	210	56.0	17
1500 pg	4	1,660	130	75.0	8
2000 pg	6	2,250	120	49.0	5
Plasma Samples		Mean pg/ml			
Female—midcycle	8	513	42	14.8	8
Female—pooled	6	145	24	9.7	17
Male—individual	6	17.4	2.8	1.1	16

From Mikhail. 1970. Steroids, 14:347.

TABLE 2

Accuracy and Reproducibility of the Estrone Method

	No. of determinations	Mean pg	Standard deviation	Standard error	Coefficient of variation (percent)
Water blank	4	14	2	1.0	14
Water + added estrone					
100 pg	4	121	15	8.0	12
200 pg	4	216	17	9.0	8
500 pg	4	530	85	43.0	16
1000 pg	3	1,030	140	80.0	13
Plasma Samples		Mean pg/ml			
Female—midcycle	8	338	36	13.0	11
Female—pooled	7	100	15	6.0	15
Male—individual	6	74	13	6.0	18

From Mikhail. 1970. Steroids, 14:345.

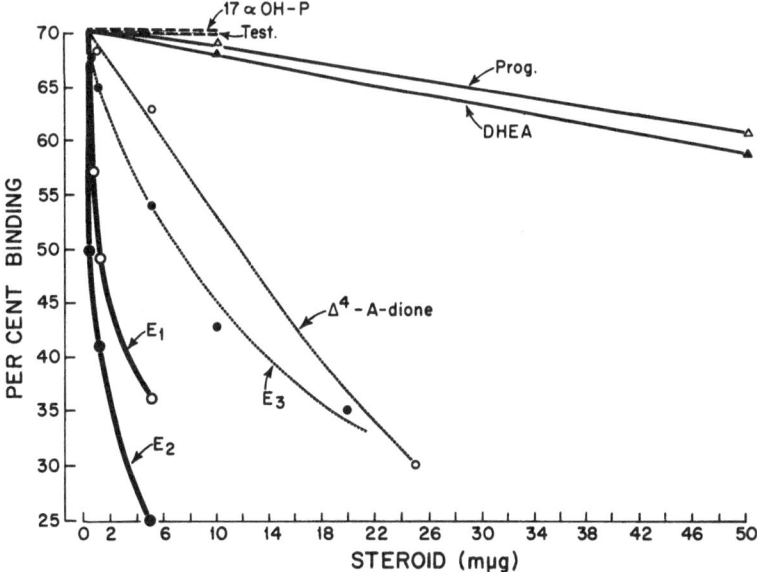

Fig. 7. Cross-reaction of various steroids with estradiol antibodies.

made (Tables 1 and 2). The coefficient of variation was 8 to 18 percent for estrone and 4 to 17 percent for estradiol.

In order to examine the specificity of the method, a number of neutral and phenolic steroids were tested for their ability to displace ^{3}H-estradiol from the antibody reagent (Fig. 7). The three estrogens competed to various degrees in this system. With the exception of androstenedione, the cross-reaction of the neutral steroids tested was negligible (less than 0.6 percent). The specificity of the method was further enhanced by the use of column chromatography which effectively separated estrone, estradiol, and estriol, in addition to separating the three estrogens from all the neutral steroids tested.

DISCUSSION

The assay method developed in our laboratory represents a simple, accurate, and practical means for the determination of plasma estrogens. Both estrone and estradiol can be measured in 16 plasma samples by one person in less than 2 days. It should be stressed, however, that the meticulous cleaning of glassware and the use of high-grade solvents are essential in order to minimize the blank of the method.

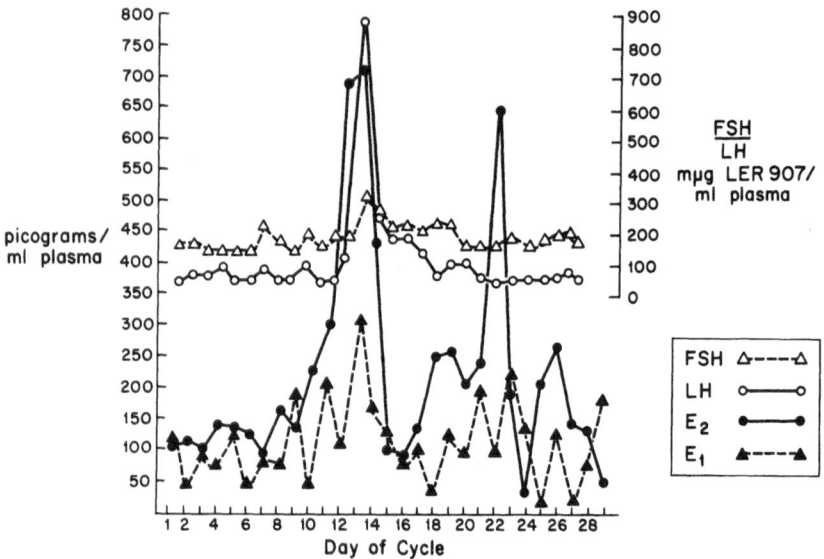

Fig. 8. Gonadotropins and estrogens in plasma during the normal menstrual cycle.

Because of the stability of the polymerized antiserum, large volumes are usually prepared and stored. In this way, polymerization of antisera is done only once every 3 to 6 months. The step of pipetting the tracer into individual reaction tubes, though used in other radioimmunoassay procedures (Midgley et al., 1969; Abraham, 1969), has been eliminated because the reagent used in our method already contains the tracer.

Baird and Guevara (1969), using a double isotope method (Baird, 1968), measured the circulating levels of estrone and estradiol during the menstrual cycle, but the report did not include a complete cycle in a single individual. We have studied the daily concentrations of circulating FSH, LH, estrone, and estradiol throughout the menstrual cycle, e.g., see Figure 8. A midcycle peak of estradiol of 1 or 2 days duration, occurring immediately prior to or coinciding with the LH peak, was detected in all the cycles studied. The levels of estradiol during the luteal phase of the cycle were higher than in the proliferative phase. No definitive midcycle peak of estrone could be detected. Moreover, there was no consistent pattern for circulating estrone in the cycles studied. This may be due in part to factors influencing the extragonadal sources of estrone (MacDonald et al., 1967). Further investigations, including the simultaneous determination of both estrone and estradiol in different physiologic and pathologic states, may shed more light on the possible mutual or independent roles of these two potent estrogens.

REFERENCES

Abraham, G. E. 1969. Solid-phase radioimmunoassay of estradiol-17β. J. Clin. Endocr., 29:866–870.

Avrameas, S., and T. Ternynck. 1967. Biologically active water-insoluble protein polymers. J. Biol. Chem., 242:1651–1659.

Baird, D. T. 1968. A method for the measurement of estrone and estradiol-17β in peripheral human blood and other biological fluids using ³⁵S-pipsyl chloride. J. Clin. Endocr., 28:244–258.

———— and A. Guevara. 1969. Concentration of unconjugated estrone and estradiol in peripheral plasma in non-pregnant women throughout the menstrual cycle, castrate and postmenopausal women and in men. J. Clin. Endocr., 29:149–156.

Catt, K., and G. W. Tregear. 1967. Solid-phase radioimmunoassay in antibody-coated tubes. Science, 158:1570–1572.

Donini, S., I. D'Alessio, and P. Donini. 1968. Radioimmunoassay of human chorionic gonadotropin and human luteinizing hormone using insoluble antibodies. *In* Rosemberg, E., ed. Gonadotropins, 1968. Los Altos, California, Geron-X, Inc. pp. 263–272.

Ferin, M., P. E. Zimmering, and R. L. Vande Wiele. 1969. Effects of antibodies to estradiol-17β on PMS-induced ovulation in immature rats. Endocrinology, 84:893–900.

———— P. E. Zimmering, S. Lieberman, and R. L. Vande Wiele. 1968. Inactivation of the biological effects of exogenous and endogenous estrogens by antibodies to 17β-estradiol. Endocrinology, 83:565–571.

MacDonald, P. C., R. P. Rombaut, and P. K. Siiteri. 1967. Plasma precursors of estrogen. I. Extent of conversion of plasma Δ⁴-androstenedione to estrone in normal males and non-pregnant normal, castrate and adrenalectomized females. J. Clin. Endocr., 27:1103–1111.

Midgley, A. R., Jr., G. D. Niswender, and J. Sri Ram. 1969. Hapten-radioimmunoassay: A general procedure for the estimation of steroidal and other haptenic substances. Steroids, 13:731–737.

Neill, J. D., E. D. B. Johansson, J. K. Datta, and E. Knobil. 1967. Relationship between the plasma levels of luteinizing hormone and progesterone during the normal menstrual cycle. J. Clin. Endocr., 37:1167–1173.

Niswender, G. D., and A. R. Midgley, Jr. 1969. Hapten-radioimmunoassay of testosterone. *In* Program of the Endocrine Society, Abstract No. 22.

DISCUSSION

M. Lipsett. Thank you, Dr. Mikhail. I would like to make one comment. From a variety of studies with several protein-binding methods, it does seem to be important to use steroid blank plasma rather than water, since in a particular method, one cannot predict whether the plasma blank will make a difference or not. I wonder if it might not be appropriate for the NIH, for example, in addition to distributing tritiated and ^{14}C steroids, to accumulate a pool of steroid blank plasma which would be available to investigators. Many of us have trouble getting plasma from adrenalectomized-gonadectomized subjects when it is needed for this sort of study.

G. MIKHAIL. I think this is a plausible idea. However, occasionally we were fortunate to have some postmenopausal blood samples that gave readings anywhere from 0 to 8 pg, so we assumed that this would tell us what blanks we were dealing with and that they were not contributing significantly to the physiologic levels reported in these studies.

N. MOUDGAL. In regard to polymerization with ethyl chloroformate, I would like to know whether you will lose any antibody activity by polymerizing.

G. MIKHAIL. Dr. Abraham is able to do his assay with a dilution of 1:20,000, but using the same antisera we cannot go over 1:600. I do not think the comparison is appropriate, however, since the binding in our method may be as high as 96 percent. We think that somewhere in the processing of the antisera we are losing some antibody. Just a few weeks ago we processed one antiserum and managed to get an antibody titer up to 1:10,000 with a binding of 60 to 70 percent. It is quite possible that, during the several procedures between obtaining the antibody and completion of the polymerization, we may be removing some of the antibody and therefore lowering the titer. This is especially possible after the exhaustive washes of the polymerized antiserum.

L. GOODFRIEND. In our laboratories, we used the Avrameas technique with slight modification for quantitative immunoadsorption of gamma-G globulin. We found no loss of antibody activity on polymerization. The difficulty we had in the original Avrameas technique was too high a nonspecific adsorption of the gamma globulin that we were interested in adsorbing. We found that by polymerizing normal serum and by using shorter incubation times, we could cut the nonspecific adsorption to about 5 to 10 percent. Did you employ normal serum at the same dilution, and, if so, how much steroid was bound by this polymerized normal serum?

G. MIKHAIL. We did not try to polymerize plain serum but this could be done very easily. We checked indirectly by processing antiserum for other steroids, namely testosterone, and found no cross-reaction. There was a previous question which asked whether, in the radioimmunoassay of steroids, a displacement of tracer from the antibody sites really occurred or whether the tracer just hooked to the sites that are available after the cold material was added. I think our method which utilizes the reverse, i.e., the tracer added to the antibody and the cold standards then used to displace the antiserum, clarifies that point.

A. SEHON.   There were a number of people who discussed, yesterday and today, the question of irreversibility of binding of hydrophobic steroids to antibodies, and who stated that equilibrium constants are very high. In your work you are using the insolubilized antibody instead of attaching it to the surface and so are making a polymer which is not suspended. Do you reuse this polymer again?

G. MIKHAIL.   No, for a number of reasons. First, the protein-fraction, i.e., antibody, is separated by very tight centrifugation, and it is very hard to remove it from the tube by just a water solvent. We have to measure residual radioactivity by washing with methanol and this would ruin the polymer. However, if we can retrieve the antiserum, we are not really aware of the number of counts or the titer of the antiserum. It would not serve as an ideal condition for reuse, and is really not necessary because of the small amount of antibody used. However, your point is well taken and this should be done just on an experimental basis.

A. SEHON.   I think this was for clarification of the methodology. If you cannot reuse your antiserum, are you not losing antibodies by making these immunosolvents, since a lot of antibody sites will be embedded into the polymer and not accessible to the hapten which you are trying to measure. In other words, you have particles of polymeric material floating around. Some of the antibody active sites are inside the matrix and may not be accessible to estradiol molecules which you are binding to the antibody active site. Therefore, the capacity of your immunosolvent in principle should be less than the capacity of the plastic coating procedure; so, in terms of making antibodies, you need a larger amount of antibody to run a number of assays than the other people who can dilute 1:50,000 or so.

G. MIKHAIL.   Yes, and in answer to this I can say the following: We feel that the thorough homogenization of polymerized antiserum obviates to a degree the phenomenon you described of trapping the active sites within a large polymer. On the other hand, your point might be valid as seen when we compare the two assays in terms of the potency of the antibody, except for the incidental finding, where processing the same antiserum yielded antibody with good titers at 10,000 or 20,000 dilution. Also, you must remember we have chosen to start with a binding of 80 percent, whereas if we want to start with a binding of 60 or 40 percent, we can comfortably work within a range of 1:2,000. Even working with a range of 1:450, all the experiments have utilized a total of only 6 or 7 ml of antiserum during a 6- or 7-month period; so, unless the material becomes really scarce and expensive, I do not think this is the limiting factor. However, we are trying to work on increasing the antibody titer, not for the sake of economy, but because a higher dilution might solve some of the problems we are encountering.

A. SEHON. Mr. Chairman, if I may make some final comments and suggestions to the people who are working in this field, there is a very simple solvent which can be prepared by adding ethylene maleic anhydride polymer to the antibody solution. This can be obtained from Monsanto without charge. You just leave it in the cold room with the steroid to produce a polymer. It copolymerizes the gamma globulin antibody by the reaction with the maleic anhydride groups.

E. KNOBIL. Those of us who work with relatively small experimental animals, in our instance the rhesus monkey, are very limited by the amount of plasma available to us, especially if we want to do serial measurements and, in this instance, sensitivity becomes of prime importance. Now using the same antiserum that you have used, Dr. Ferin's antibody, at a dilution of 1:90,000, Dr. Hotkiss in our laboratory has devised a radioimmunoassay for estradiol which has a sensitivity of 5 pg, and this permits us to measure estradiol and estrone reliably in 200-lambda aliquots of peripheral plasma. One of the reasons we have been able to achieve this sensitivity is the application of the discontinuous trace addition idea of Dr. Midgley. While it is perfectly true that cold material can displace tracer from the antibody, a greater sensitivity is achieved if the tracer is added later. The procedure used in our laboratory is to add the cold material first, followed by the antibody, and to incubate the mixture at room temperature for 30 minutes. The tracer is then added and the incubation is continued in the cold for an additional 16 to 20 hours. To separate the bound from free estradiol we use Dextran-coated charcoal and a phosphate buffer system which contains 1 percent gelatin. This procedure results reliably in a standard curve as shown in Figure 1 below.

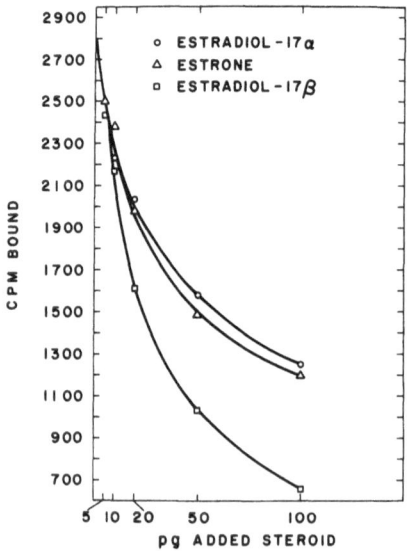

7

SOLID-PHASE RADIOIMMUNOASSAY
OF STEROIDS

Stephen A. Tillson, Ian H. Thorneycroft,
Guy E. Abraham,* Rex J. Scaramuzzi, Burton V. Caldwell
Worcester Foundation for Experimental Biology
Shrewsbury, Massachusetts

INTRODUCTION

There have been several procedures reported which offer the new investigator interested in developing a radioimmunoassay for steroid hormones a choice of methods for separating the free from bound steroid. Midgley et al. (1969) have described a means for accomplishing separation, based on precipitation of bound antibody-steroid with a second antibody. This separation usually requires incubation for several days. Mikhail et al. (1970) separate free from bound estradiol by polymerizing the antibody, but this adds a high-speed centrifugation step. The recently described solid-phase system for estradiol (Abraham, 1969; Abraham and Odell, 1970) would appear to offer many advantages over the above procedures, particularly the unique feature of accomplishing the equilibration and the separation of free from bound steroid in a single step. It will be the principal aim of this paper to describe in detail the several essential criteria which must be examined for each antiserum, central to its use in the development of new methods for the radioimmunoassay of

This work was supported by training grant 5-T01-AMO 5564-13 from the National Institute of Arthritis and Metabolic Diseases, USPHS, administered by Fernand C. Péron.
* Present address: Division of Endocrinology, Harbor General Hospital, Torrance, California.

steroids. Chemical, immunologic, and endocrinologic aspects of steroid-protein conjugates have been described by Lieberman et al. (1959). Pressman and Grossberg (1968, 1970) have discussed chemical and structural concepts which are involved in antibody-antigen interactions. However, the effects of certain physicochemical factors, such as ionic strength, hydrogen ion concentration, and temperature, on potential radioimmunoassay systems for progesterone and testosterone have not been previously examined in detail and will be described below as they apply to the solid-phase assay of these hormones.

ANTIBODY SOURCE

The anti-steroid antibodies used in this study were obtained from sheep at the Worcester Foundation, with the exception of an antiprogesterone antibody, also from sheep, which was kindly supplied to us by Drs. Ferin and Vande Wiele. The antigens used were testosterone-17- and estradiol-17-hemisuccinates, and progesterone-20-oxime *o*-carboxy-methyl derivatives, all of which were linked to purified bovine serum albumin. Details of the preparation and purification of these antisera are given elsewhere in this symposium (Thorneycroft et al., 1970).

COATING OF ANTIBODY TO POLYSTYRENE TUBES

Catt and Tregear (1967) reported a procedure utilizing the ability of the antibody to adsorb to polymer surfaces lacking defined reactive groups and based on the fact that antibodies directed against peptide hormones would bind to polypropylene and polystyrene tubes. Abraham (1969) applied this technique to radioimmunoassay of estradiol-17β. In our tube-binding studies, an antibody to estradiol-17β was obtained from sheep serum and labeled with [125]I. Fifteen micrograms of antisera to estradiol-17β were added to the reaction vessel with I μl of ^{125}I and 50 μg of Chloramine T (Greenwood et al., 1963). The antibody was reacted for 2 minutes and the oxidation reaction was stopped by addition of 1.25 mg sodium metabisulphite. The organic-bound iodine was separated from the unreacted substances by column chromatography using Sephadex G-75 and 0.01 M phosphate buffer in 0.9 percent saline. One-half-milliliter fractions were collected and counted on a γ-spectrometer. The tube with maximum activity in the first peak was used for the coating experiment. Trace amounts (60,000 cpm) of ^{125}I-antibody to estradiol-17β (SA 26.1 μc/μg) were added to dilutions of antibody to estradiol-17β of 1:500, 1:5,000, and 1:10,000. Figure 1 shows the results

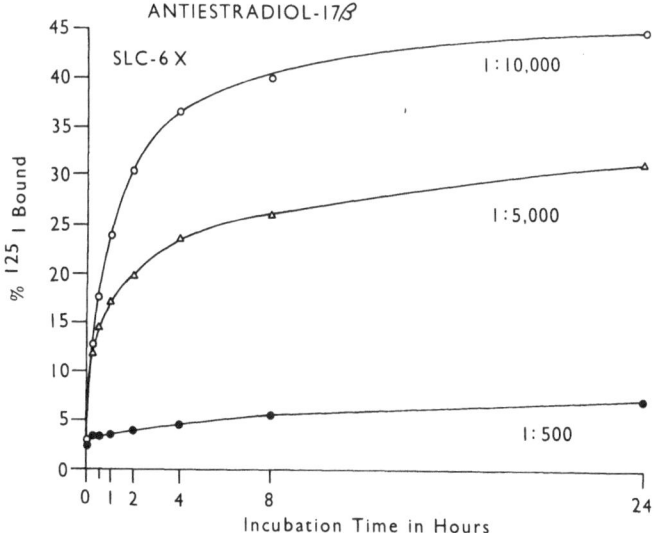

Fig. 1. The effect of dilution of antisera on the time of coating of the antibody to polystyrene tubes.

obtained when polystyrene tubes were incubated at 23°C in pH 9.6 barbital buffer. The lower the dilution of antisera the less radioactivity bound, due to the ratio of labeled to unlabeled antibody, and therefore the more unlabeled mass coated. As the concentration of unlabeled mass decreased, a higher percentage of radioactive mass coated. There was an increased binding of the antiserum to the tube as the duration of coating increased. These data are consistent with the data reported by Catt (1969).

CONDITIONS AFFECTING THE BINDING OF STEROIDS TO ANTIBODIES

Temperature

The effect of temperature may be related to the free energy of antigen-antibody reaction and the stability of the protein. In Table 1, the optimum temperature can be seen for antibody directed against estradiol-17β. At 37°C the binding of the antibody decreased with incubation time. Maximum binding occurred at 4°C between 8 and 24 hours with antisera to estradiol-17β and progesterone. Testosterone bound maximally at 4°C between 4 and 8 hours. Pressman et al. (1961a) showed

TABLE 1

Optimum Conditions for Measuring Estradiol, Progesterone, and Testosterone by Solid-Phase Radioimmunoassay Procedures

Antisera	Tube coating conditions	Incubation conditions	pH range	Molarity
Estradiol SLC-6X	8-24 hr at 4°C pH 9.6-10.2	8-24 hr at 4°C	6.8-7.2	0.1M phosphate buffer
Progesterone R-1	8-24 hr at 4°C pH 9.6-10.2	8-24 hr at 4°C	5.8-7.6	2.0M (NaCl) in 0.1M phosphate buffer
Testosterone 84-9B	8-24 hr at 4°C pH 9.6-10.2	4-8 hr at 4°C	5.8-6.8	0.1M phosphate buffer

increased binding of anti-p-azobenzoate antibody with decreasing temperature and that enthalpy accounted for approximately 60 percent of the free energy change. Similar temperature effects have been obtained from α_1-acid glycoproteins (Ganguly et al., 1967; Ganguly and Westphal, 1968). Not all antisera behave in the same manner, however, since there are examples of estradiol-17β antisera which bind better at 23°C (Jiang and Ryan, 1969; Abraham and Odell, 1970). Therefore, each antiserum should be tested for temperature effects.

pH

Pressman et al. (1961b) reports that anti-p-azobenzoate antibody shows a decrease in binding with increasing pH (pH 8 to 10), which was attributed to the loss of a proton from the active site at the higher pH values. This also was true for antibodies directed against compounds with neutral and acidic groups, and indicated that OH groups were present in the sites of all the antibodies they tested. When the pH value for antibodies against acidic group antigens was below pH 5, there was a decreased combination with the specific hapten. This decreased binding was thought to be due to protonation of an essential carboxylate group in the active site. The carboxylate group was present only in the antibody with an acidic hapten (Pressman and Grossberg, 1968). The reader is referred to Pressman and Grossberg (1970) for more complete and detailed information on the structural basis of antibody specificity.

The range of pH used in this study (5.8 to 8) was between the extremes reported to have an effect on binding (Pressman and Grossberg, 1968), and was considered to be the best range to run an assay system. There was approximately 7.6 percent variation in binding between pH 5.8 and pH 7.6 with the antibody directed against progesterone, and 6.8

percent variation in binding between pH 5.8 and pH 6.8 with the antibody directed against testosterone. It should be noted that there was approximately a 2.8 percent variation in binding between pH 5.8 and pH
7.6 for nonimmunized sheep serum treated in the same manner as the
antisera. It appears that the assay can be used anywhere in the pH range
tested without affecting the assay system.

Ionic Strength

The recent studies of Ganguly et al. (1967) and Ganguly and Westphal (1968) showed an increased binding in the presence of neutral salts.
This fact prompted us to determine if increasing molar salt concentration affected the binding of the hapten to the antibody. The progesterone antisera showed a threefold increase in binding with 1 M NaCl and
a fivefold increase with 2 M NaCl as compared to control values.

Testosterone antibody, on the other hand, showed approximately a
25 percent increase at 2 M NaCl over control values. Nonspecific binding
also rose slightly with increasing NaCl concentration (6.5 percent from 0
to 4 M). The conformational structure of globular proteins was apparently stabilized by NaCl and other neutral salts (Ganguly and Westphal,
1968). This may provide a better fit for the hapten-antibody interaction.
The data reported by Pressman et al. (1961a, b) and Grossberg et al.
(1962) indicated that some antibodies have a charge on the antibody-
hapten-combining site which is opposite to that of the hapten. They also
suggested that the salt ion (either positive or negative depending on the
charge of the active site) competed with the hapten for the active site
and therefore decreased hapten binding. The antibodies used in this
study were basically derived from uncharged derivatives with, for example, no free carboxylate or ammonium ions available to cause a charge in
the antibody-combining site, perhaps, explaining why there appeared to
be no competition between salt ions and the hapten.

SOLID-PHASE SYSTEM

Antisera to estradiol, testosterone, and progesterone were processed
in a manner similar to that previously reported for the estradiol-17β antibody (Abraham, 1969) and detailed in this symposium by Thorneycroft
et al. (1970). Briefly, polystyrene tubes were coated to 0.4 ml with Rivanol-treated*antisera in barbital buffer (Table 2). After removing the
coating solution the tubes were washed three times with 0.01 M phosphate buffer. The phosphate buffer was removed and varying amounts of
authentic steroid (previously dissolved in phosphate buffer) were added

TABLE 2

Assay Conditions for Solid-Phase Radioimmunoassay

ANTIBODY-COATING CONDITIONS:	0.4 ml of Rivanol-treated antisera in barbital buffer 0.07 M, pH 9.6-10.2
INCUBATION CONDITIONS:	18-24 hr at 4°C
WASHING:	3 times 0.1 M phosphate buffer 0.4 ml
ADDITION OF STANDARDS:	Standards dissolved in 0.1 M phosphate buffer are added in varying amounts and brought to 0.4 ml with phosphate buffer
ADDITION OF RADIOACTIVITY:	^{3}H-steroid 0.005 μc in 0.1 ml of 0.1 M phosphate buffer to each tube
MIXING:	Vortex mixer
INCUBATION CONDITIONS:	4-24 hr at 4°C
QUANTITATION:	Quantitative removal of buffer 10 ml toluene-base scintillator (Liquifluor-BBS-3) added. Percent bound ^{3}H-steroid calculated

to coated tubes. Additional phosphate buffer was added to appropriate tubes to attain a constant volume of 0.4 ml per tube.

To each tube was added 0.1 ml of phosphate buffer containing approximately 0.005 μc of the appropriate ^{3}H-steroid. The tubes were mixed on a vortex mixer and incubated at 4°C for at least 8 hours. The supernatant was quantitatively transferred to scintillation vials to which was added 10 ml of a toluene-base scintillation fluid. The amount of radioactivity in the vials was counted and the percent of bound ^{3}H-steroid was calculated.

Incubation Time

Incubation time in solid-phase radioimmunoassay of steroids is not as critical as with saturation analysis systems when florisil or charcoal are used for separation of free from bound steroid. In solid-phase, the separation step is independent of the hapten and therefore the equilibrium is not disturbed by separation. With double-antibody techniques, the incubation takes 5 days for binding and precipitation of the binding antibody with the second, or precipitating antibody (Midgley et al., 1969). Table 1 shows that incubation times between 4 and 24 hours are sufficient for the assay systems.

Standard Curves

Increasing amounts of unlabeled steroid displace increasing amounts of bound labeled steroid (Figs. 2, 3, and 4). Each point on the individual

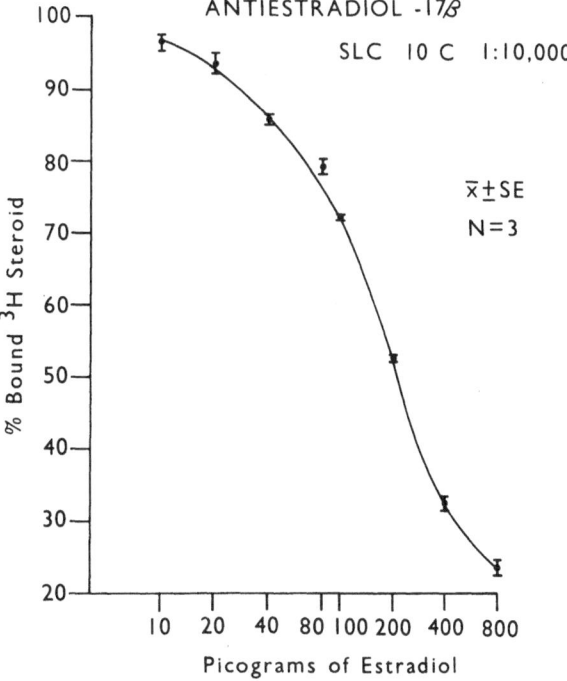

Fig. 2. Standard curve for estradiol-17β using antibodies directed against estradiol-17ß in the solid-phase system.

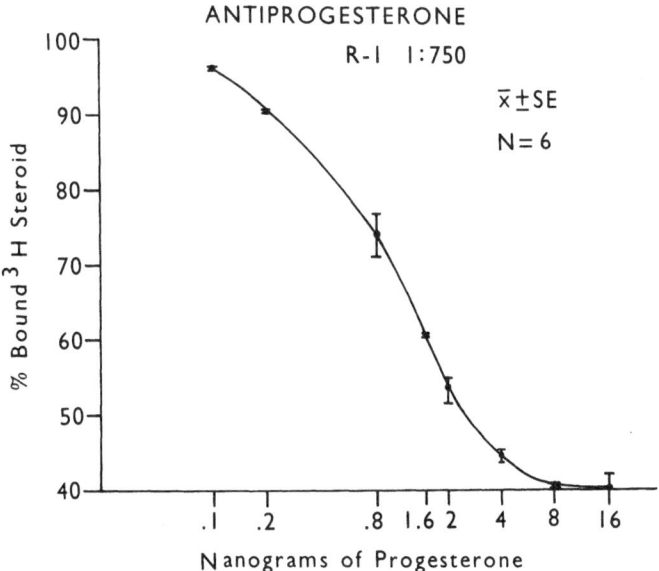

Fig. 3. Standard curve for progesterone using antibodies directed against progesterone in the solid-phase system.

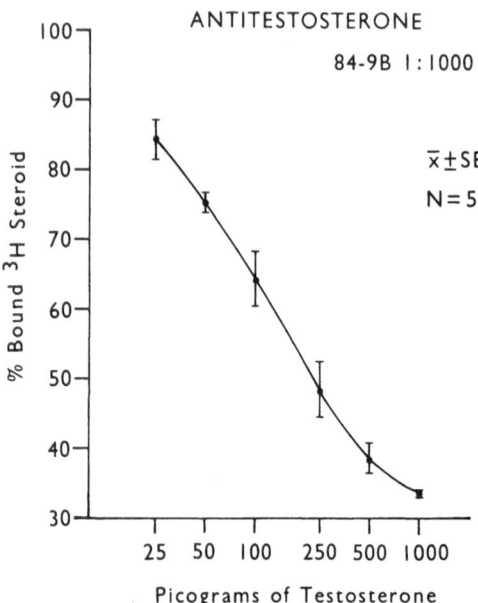

Fig. 4. Standard curve for testosterone using antibodies directed against testosterone in the solid-phase system.

standard curves represents the mean and standard error of the mean for triplicate, quadruplicate, and quintuplicate samples for estradiol-17β, progesterone, and testosterone, respectively. The coefficient of variation and linear regression equations are: 3.0 percent, $Y = 1.49 + (-0.42)$ (log X) for estradiol; 2.1 percent, $Y = 0.65 + (-0.17)$ (log X) for progesterone; and 9.0 percent, $Y = 1.31 + (-0.38)$ (log X) for testosterone. Equilibrium constants for the antibodies were calculated from a Scatchard plot, as modified by Sandberg et al. (1966). Bound and free hormone were equilibrated in the solid-phase system rather than by equilibrium dialysis. In the solid-phase system, the antibody is not, however, in true solution as it is in the equilibrium dialysis system. Therefore, the constants presented have merit only from a comparative aspect with other antibodies used in the solid-phase system. Equilibrium constants for estradiol-17β, testosterone, and progesterone were 2.9×10^{10}, 1.6×10^{9}, and 2.0×10^{8}, respectively.

Cross-Reactions

The relative affinities of other steroids tested for specific antisera (Tables 3, 4, and 5) are expressed as percent equivalents of the steroid

TABLE 3

Cross-Reactions of Various Steroids with Antiserum Directed against Estradiol-17β

Steroid tested	Cross-reaction (percent)
C^{18} Steroid	
Estradiol-17β	100.0
Estradiol-17α	80.0
Estrone	33.0
Estriol	6.0
C^{19} Steroid	
Testosterone	0.4
Epitestosterone	0.0
Androstenedione	0.0
C^{21} Steroid	
Progesterone	0.003
Cortisol	0.0009
C^{27} Steroid	
Cholesterol	0.0

specific for its antisera. The cross-reaction with estradiol-17β antisera for estradiol-17α, estrone, and estriol was 80 percent, 33 percent, and 6 percent, respectively, while the neutral steroids cross-react only slightly or not at all, the highest being testosterone at 0.4 percent. The antiserum to testosterone cross-reacted greatest with low concentrations of androstenedione and epitestosterone, and least at higher concentration of these steroids. A possible explanation for this peculiar result is that the affinity of the antibody Δ^4-3-keto steroids is extremely high, but it has a low

TABLE 4

Cross-Reactions of Various Steroids with Antiserum Directed against Progesterone

Steroid tested	Cross-reaction (percent)
C^{18} Steroid	
Estradiol-17β	0.0
C^{19} Steroid	
Testosterone	53.0
C^{21} Steroid	
Progesterone	100.0
Corticosterone	4.4
C^{27} Steroid	
Cholesterol	1.0

TABLE 5

Cross-Reactions of Various Steroids with Antiserum Directed against Testosterone

Steroid tested	Cross-reaction (percent)
C^{18} Steroid	
Estradiol-17β	0.0
C^{19} Steroid	
Testosterone	100.0
Epitestosterone	66.0
Androstenedione	145.0
C^{21} Steroid	
Progesterone	14.5
Corticosterone	14.5
C^{27} Steroid	
Cholesterol	1.0

capacity. These sites are saturated quickly while other sites on the antibody specific for other portions of the hapten show a relatively lower specificity with a larger capacity and may exclude related steroids with side chain differences (Fig. 5).

Phenolic steroids, i.e., estrogens, do not appear to bind with the antibodies directed against the neutral steroids (i.e., testosterone or progeste-

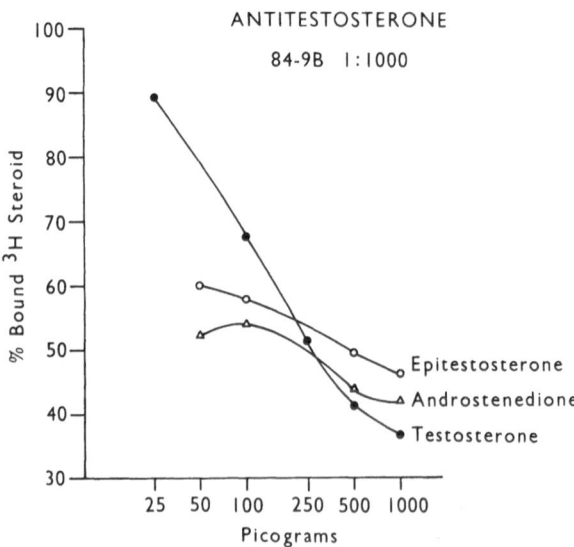

Fig. 5. Cross-reaction of androstenedione and epitestosterone, compared with testosterone, using the antibodies directed against testosterone in the solid-phase system.

rone). The data on cross-reaction point out the need for separation of the steroids from the extracted plasma before using them in the solid-phase assay system.

High cross-reactions may not always be undesirable. For example, using estrone as the hapten for anti-estradiol-17β antibody, a standard curve can be constructed (Fig. 6). The measurement of both estrone and

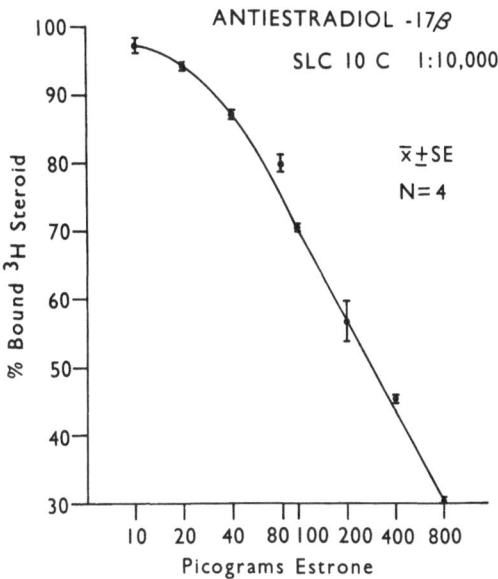

Fig. 6. Standard curve for estrone using antibodies directed against estradiol-17β in the solid-phase system.

estradiol-17β, using antisera to estradiol-17β, is now available from a single plasma sample using the separation techniques discussed at this symposium (Abraham and Odell, 1970).

THE USE OF STEROID ANTIBODIES WITH OTHER SEPARATION SYSTEMS

In Table 6 some of the methods of separation used in current assay systems are shown. The reference list is not complete and not intended to be an exhaustive list, but provides a reference where more detailed information can be found. Not all antisera are suited for solid-phase systems. For example, one antiprogesterone antiserum had approximately 30 percent binding at 1:100 dilution when tested by the solid-phase system, as

TABLE 6

Separation Methods Used in Steroid-Protein Binding Assays

Protein source	Method of separation (free from bound)	References
Plasma		
CBG, TBG, or EBG	a. Florisil	Murphy, 1967; Neill et al., 1967
	b. Ammonium sulfate	Mayes and Nugent, 1968; Maeda et al., 1969
	c. Sephadex	Kato and Horton, 1968; Yoshimi and Lipsett, 1968
	d. Fuller's earth	Murphy, 1967
	e. Charcoal-dextran	Horton, et al., 1967; Murphy, 1967; Rosenfield et al., 1969
γ-Globulins	a. Solid phase	Abraham, 1969; Tillson et al., 1970
	b. Polymerization	Mikhail and Ferin, 1970
	c. Double antibody	Midgley et al., 1969
	d. Florisil	Tillson et al., 1970
	e. Charcoal-dextran	Jiang and Ryan, 1969
	f. Dowex-1	Jiang and Ryan, 1969
Other tissues		
Soluble uterine macromolecule	a. Charcoal-dextran	Korenman, 1968

compared to 60 percent binding when used in a saturation-analysis system with florisil as an adsorbent of free steroid. Table 7 shows a comparison of Rivanol-treated antiprogesterone antisera compared to unstressed dog plasma. The advantage of using an antiserum to a specific hormone, as opposed to other serum proteins, is that essentially a more purified and constant source of protein may be available which would make it

TABLE 7

A Comparison of Progesterone Antisera and Nonimmunized Plasma Proteins in a Saturation Analysis System Using Florisil for Separation of Bound from Free Steroid

Anti-progesterone[a]		Dog plasma[b]	
ng added	cpm bound	ng added	cpm bound
0.00	1880	0.0	1675
0.25	1686	0.2	1580
0.50	1561	0.4	1520
1.00	1319	0.6	1440
2.50	1174	1.0	1310
5.00	1072		
10.00	826		

[a]Sheep 83 antisera-dilution 1:100.
[b]Data extrapolated from Neill et al. 1967. Plasma-dilution 1:40 (2.5%).

possible to provide a standardized assay to laboratories. In addition, it may be possible to measure a greater range of steroid hormones. Yoshimi and Lipsett (1968) reported a sensitivity of 0.1 ng of progesterone with a range from 0.1 to 3 ng at a 1:100 dilution of human plasma.

VALIDITY OF THE ASSAY

The most stringent test of an assay system is to show that hormone recovered from plasma behaves the same as authentic standards. In accordance with the procedure below, 20 to 400 pg of authentic estradiol-17β were added to 1 ml of adrenalectomized-ovariectomized

EXTRACTION PROCEDURE FOR ESTRADIOL-17β

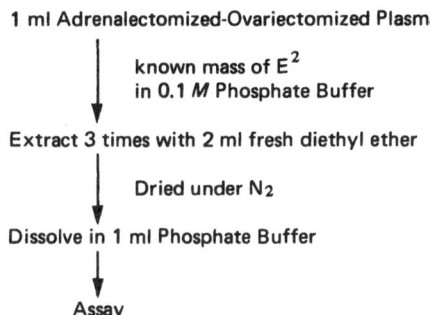

1 ml Adrenalectomized-Ovariectomized Plasma

known mass of E^2
in 0.1 M Phosphate Buffer

Extract 3 times with 2 ml fresh diethyl ether

Dried under N_2

Dissolve in 1 ml Phosphate Buffer

Assay

sheep plasma. The samples were extracted three times with 2 ml of fresh diethyl ether. The pooled ether was evaporated, the residue dissolved in 1 ml of phosphate buffer, and 0.4 ml used in the assay as previously described. In addition, authentic estradiol-17β was added to water in amounts ranging from 20 to 240 pg. These samples were extracted three

TABLE 8
Recovery of Estradiol-17β from Plasma or Water[a]

Estradiol added	Estradiol recovered from plasma	Estradiol recovered from water
(pg)	(pg)	(pg)
400	376.6 ± 23.3[b]	—
240	277.5 ± 16.6	247.9 ± 20.7[b]
160	172.6 ± 9.9	154.6 ± 3.2
80	68.0 ± 11.0	70.8 ± 1.7
40	20.5 ± 10.4	34.0 ± 5.3
20	11.5 ± 3.0	24.4 ± 12.2

[a] $n = 3$.
[b] Mean ± standard deviation.

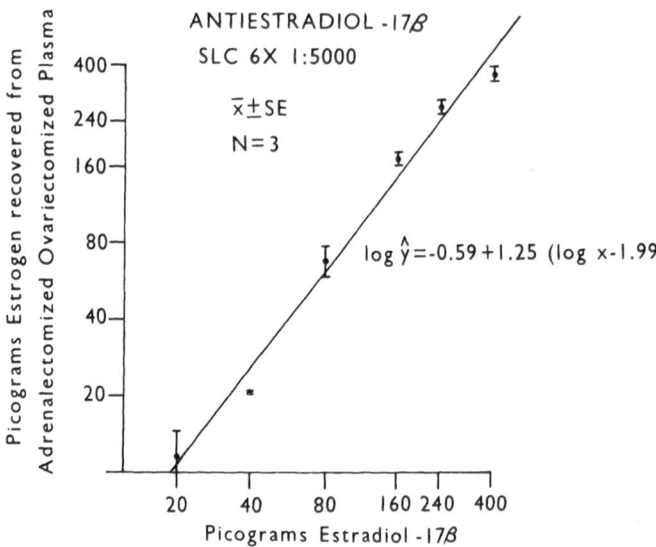

Fig. 7. Regression line calculated for estradiol-17β extracted from plasma.

times with 2 ml of fresh diethyl ether. The pooled ether was evaporated, the residue dissolved in 1.0 ml of phosphate buffer, and 0.4 ml used in the assay as previously described. In addition, authentic estradiol-17β was added to water in amounts ranging from 20 to 240 pg. These samples were extracted in the same way as the plasma samples and run in the assay system. The means and standard deviation are presented in Table 8. Generally, the assay tends to overestimate at the higher concentration of steroid and underestimate at the lower concentration of steroid. This perhaps causes the greatest concern in using the assay for routine measurement. When the data are analyzed by least squares fit for linear regression (Fig. 7), they confirm the trends shown in Table 8. The other antibodies have not yet been subjected to the same test as the antibody to estradiol. Work is in progress to test these systems.

SUMMARY

Information obtained from studies on pH, temperature, and ionic strength was used to construct standard curves and estimate equilibrium constants. The interaction of the antibody with steroids other than the haptenic steroid for the antibody production was tested. So far, antibodies tested in our laboratory have not been specific for a particular steroid without some minor cross-reactions with structurally similar steroids. The use of the antibody in lieu of other plasma globulins has also been investigated using a typical saturation-analysis system. Antibodies to progesterone appeared to be comparable, if not better than other plasma proteins, in their ability to bind and allow displacement of labeled steroid with increasing mass of unlabeled steroid. Finally, the validity of the method, and perhaps the most stringent test, is to extract known amounts of steroid from plasma and compare the mass recovered to the mass of steroid added. By no means are the data complete; however, enough information is available to indicate that antibodies are useful for steroid assay systems.

Acknowledgment

The authors wish to acknowledge Dr. John A. McCracken for providing and maintaining the sheep used in this study.

REFERENCES

Abraham, G. E. 1969. Solid-phase radioimmunoassay of estradiol-17β. J. Clin. Endocr., 29:866–870.

―――― and W. D. Odell. Solid-phase radioimmunoassay of serum estradiol-17β: A semi-automated approach. 1970. *In* Péron, F. G., and B. V. Caldwell, eds. Immunologic Methods in Steroid Determination. New York, Appleton-Century-Crofts.

Catt, K. J. 1969. *In* Margaulies, M., ed. Protein and Polypeptide Hormones. New York, Excerpta Medica Foundation, Part 3, pp. 639–642.

―――― and G. W. Tregear. 1967. Solid-phase radioimmunoassay in antibody-coated tubes. Science, 158:1570–1572.

Ganguly, M., and U. Westphal. 1968. Steroid-protein interactions. XVII. Influence of solvent environment on interaction between α_1 acid glycoproteins and progesterone. J. Biol. Chem., 243:6130–6139.

―――― R. H. Carneghan, and U. Westphal. 1967. Steroid-protein interactions. XIV. Interaction between human α_1 acid glycoprotein and progesterone. Biochemistry (Wash.), 6:2803–2814.

Greenwood, F. C., W. M. Hunter, and J. S. Glover. 1963. The preparations of I^{131}-labeled human growth hormone of high specific radioactivity. Biochem. J., 89:114–123.

Grossberg, A. L., C. C. Chen, L. Rendina, and D. Pressman. 1962. Specific cation effects with antibody to a hapten with a positive charge. J. Immun., 88:600–603.

Horton, R., T. Kato, and R. Sherins. 1967. A rapid method for the estimation of testosterone in male plasma. Steroids, 10:245–256.

Jiang, N. S., and R. J. Ryan. 1969. Radioimmunoassay for estrogens: A preliminary communication. Mayo Clin. Proc., 44:461–465.

Kato, T., and R. Horton. 1968. A rapid method for the estimation of testosterone in female plasma. Steroids, 12:631–650.

Korenman, S. G. 1968. Radio-ligand binding assay of specific estrogens using a soluble uterine macromolecule. J. Clin. Endocr., 28:127–130.

Lieberman, S., B. F. Erlanger, S. M. Beiser, and F. J. Agate, Jr. 1959. Steroid-protein conjugates: Their chemical immunochemical, and endocrinology properties. Recent Progr. Hormone Res., 15:165–200.

Maeda, R., M. Okamoto, L. C. Wegienka, and P. H. Forsham. 1969. A clinically useful method for plasma testosterone determination. Steroids, 13:83–99.

Mayes, D., and C. A. Nugent. 1968. Determination of plasma testosterone by the use of competitive protein binding. J. Clin. Endocr., 28:1169–1176.

Midgley, A. R., Jr., G. D. Niswender, and J. S. Ram. 1969. Hapten-radioimmunoassay: A general procedure for the estimation of standard and other haptenic substances. Steroids, 13:731–737.

Mikhail, G., C. Wu, M. Ferin, and R. L. Vande Wiele. 1970. Radioimmunoassay of plasma estrogens: Use of polymerized antibodies. In Péron, F. G., and Caldwell, B. V., eds. Immunologic Methods in Steroid Determination. New York, Appleton-Century-Crofts.

Murphy, B. E. P. 1967. Some studies of the protein-binding steroids and their application to the routine micro and ultramicro measurements of various steroids in body fluids by competitive protein-binding radioassay. J. Clin. Endocr., 27:973–990.

Neill, J. D., E. D. B. Johansson, J. K. Datta, and E. Knobil. 1967. Relationship between the plasma levels of luteinizing hormone and progesterone during the normal menstrual cycle. J. Clin. Endocr., 27:1167–1173.

Pressman, D., and A. L. Grossberg. 1968. The Structural Basis of Antibody Specificity. New York, W. A. Benjamin, Inc.

——— and A. L. Grossberg. 1970. Structural basis of antibody specificity. In Péron, F. G., and Caldwell, B. V., eds. Immunologic Methods in Steroid Determination. New York, Appleton-Century-Crofts.

——— A. Nisonoff, and G. Radzimski. 1961a. Specific anion effects with antibenzoate antibody. J. Immun., 86:35–41.

———A. Nisonoff, G. Radzimski, and A. Shaw. 1961b. Nature of the active site of antibenzoate antibodies: Further evidence for the presence of tyrosine. J. Immun., 86:489–495.

Rosenfield, R. L., W. R. Eberlein, and A. M. Bongiovanni. 1969. Measurement of plasma testosterone by means of competitive protein binding analysis. J. Clin. Endocr., 29:854–859.

Sandberg, A. A., H. Rosenthal, S. L. Schneider, and W. R. Slaunwhite, Jr. 1966. Protein-steroid interactions and their role in the transport and metabolism of steroids. In Pincus, G., T. Nakao, and J. F. Tait, eds. Steroid Dynamics. New York, Academic Press, Inc., pp. 1–62.

Thorneycroft, I. H., S. A. Tillson, G. E. Abraham, R. J. Scaramuzzi, and B. V. Caldwell. 1970. Preparation and purification of antibodies to steroids. *In* Péron, F. G., and Caldwell, B. V., eds. Immunologic Methods in Steroid Determination. New York, Appleton-Century-Crofts.

Yoshimi, T., and M. B. Lipsett. 1968. The measurement of plasma progesterone. Steroids, 11:527–540.

DISCUSSION

N. Jiang. I would like to take this opportunity to report some of the results we have obtained with a radioimmunoassay for estrogen at the Mayo Clinic. In today's sessions we have heard about solid-phase radioimmunoassays and radioimmunoassay by polymerization of the antibody. In both systems the separation of bound and free hormone is achieved either by polymerizing the antibody, and hence changing the bound hormone to an insoluble form, or by coating the antibody, and hence retaining the bound hormone on the wall of a plastic tube, leaving the free hormone in solution. I have been working with a system which removes the free hormone with an adsorbent, leaving the antibody-bound hormone in solution. An aliquot of the supernatant solution is counted to quantitate the bound hormone. I tried various adsorbents and found two that gave consistent and satisfactory results. They are Dowex-1 ion exchange resin in the chloride form and dextran-coated charcoal pretreated with 3.5 percent serum. Fig. 1 shows the elution profile of triti-

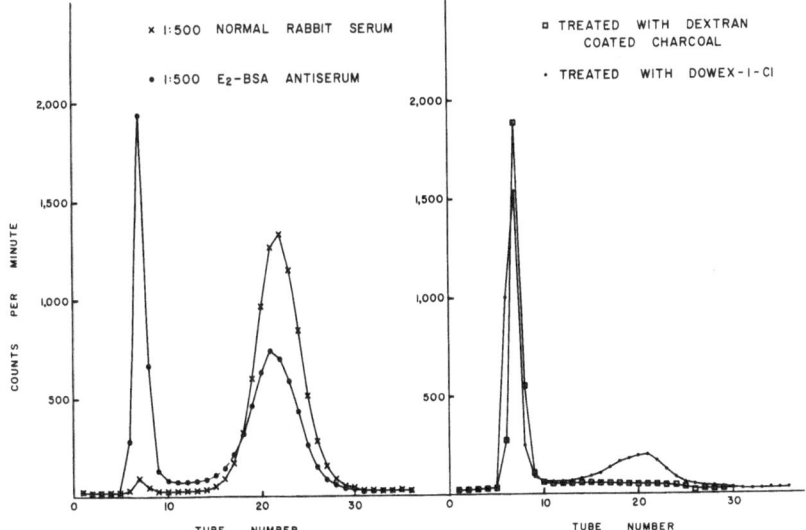

Fig. 1. The elution profile of tritiated estradiol from a Sephadex G-75 column, before and after treatment with dextran-coated charcoal or Dowex-1-Cl.

um-labeled estradiol from a 1.4 by 17-cm Sephadex G-75 column. The curves on the left show that in the presence of E$_2$-BSA antiserum (solid circles), at a 1:500 dilution, a peak of radioactivity is eluted at the void volume (tube 7) of the column, which means that the isotope is bound to a large molecule. A second peak, which is the free estradiol, occurs at tube 23. If the E$_2$-BSA antiserum is replaced by normal rabbit serum at the same dilution (x - x), only an insignificant amount of radioactivity is eluted at the void volume and all the counts are recovered as free estradiol. The curves on the right show the same incubation mixture with E$_2$-BSA antiserum, treated with 100 mg of Dowex-1-chloride (solid circles) or 25 mg of dextran-coated charcoal pretreated with 3.5 percent serum (open squares). In the Dowex-1-chloride-treated mixture, there was always a small amount of radioactivity equivalent to 10 percent of the total counts present in the mixture, remaining as free estradiol. This small, free-estradiol peak is also present in the control mixture where normal rabbit serum is used. However, in the mixture treated with dextran-coated charcoal, the free-estradiol peak is completely eliminated. The recovery of bound hormone in the supernatant is from 95 to 100 percent in both cases. If an appropriate blank value is subtracted, the Dowex-1-chloride resin gives the same results as those obtained with the dextran-coated charcoal. If the dextran-coated charcoal is not pretreated with 3.5 percent serum, all the radioactivity, bound and free, is adsorbed by the charcoal. The pretreatment with 3.5 percent serum is essential.

Figure 2 shows the results obtained with our system. As far as specificity of the antiserum is concerned, I am afraid I can add very little, if

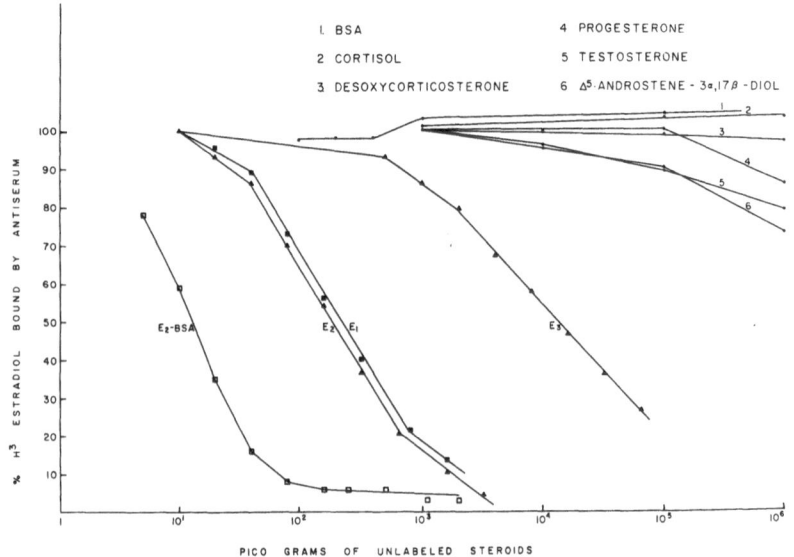

Fig. 2. Standard curve for estradiol-17β showing cross-reactions with other steroids and BSA.

anything, to what we have learned this morning. Our antiserum cannot differentiate E_1 and E_2; some of the steroids tested begin to show interference at 10^5 and 10^6 pg which is 10,000 times the amount of E_1 and E_2 required to cause significant displacement. To answer a question raised this morning concerning the necessity of adsorbing antiserum with BSA, it does not seem to be necessary with our system. Curve no. 1 shows that 10^5 pg of BSA did not displace labeled E_2. It is interesting that E_2-BSA, the original antigen, as we would have expected, replaced labeled E_2 very efficiently.

S. TILLSON.   How much dissociation of the bound steroid do you think occurs in this column-separation system? Yoshimi and Lipsett (1968) have reported competition with blood proteins and Sephadex for tritiated progesterone. We have seen similar results when we run the antibody through a 1.5 cm by 25 cm Sephadex G-100 column.

N. JIANG.   I do not know. This is a short 17-cm column. The whole operation can be finished in 5 minutes. We also run our column at 4°C in order to prevent the reverse reaction of the binding, if there is any.

W. D. ODELL.   My first question concerns the pH and molarity effects on the antisera. Did you study only one antiserum in each category or did your data come from a series of antisera?

S. TILLSON.   The data came from one antiserum for each steroid.

W. ODELL.   Can you tell us then if you have any more extensive experience to indicate whether these effects are characteristic of a particular immunogen that the antibody is directed against, or whether it just happens to be that one antiserum that you checked?

S. TILLSON.   We are in the process of testing another antiserum for each steroid but the results are not conclusive; therefore, I cannot comment on other antisera.

W. ODELL.   It is likely then, that the effects of pH and molarity relate only to the antiserum. Antisera directed against HCG show varied effects of molarity and other parameters in incubation mixtures. Your studies point out the wisdom of studying in detail many aspects of any antiserum to be used for assay purposes.

The second question I wanted to ask you: What was the cross-reaction of 17-hydroxyprogesterone in your assay for progesterone?

S. TILLSON.   We have not done that, mainly because we plan on separating. Hence, no extensive cross-reaction studies have been carried out.

W. ODELL.   How many animals did you immunize with each of these complexed antigens, what was your rate of success in each case, and what species did you use?

S. TILLSON.   We immunized two sheep each for testosterone, progesterone, and estradiol. With testosterone and progesterone we had a 50 percent success rate.

W. ODELL.   Did the other ones give no titer?

S. TILLSON.   The other testosterone and progesterone antisera were very similar in response, in that we found very low titers. The estradiol animals were both very successful. There may be a difference in antibody response for neutral versus phenolic steroids in sheep. We have immunized these animals repetitively every month for 9 months for all the steroids we injected. I am not sure about the antiserum directed against progesterone, the one obtained from the Columbia group, although I understand that this animal has been injected in a similar manner.

W. ODELL.   May I direct this question to Dr. Jiang: It was not clear from what you said whether the antiserum that you used was one you prepared yourself, or one you obtained from another group.

N. JIANG.   We used the antiserum which we ourselves obtained from rabbits.

W. ODELL.   Then, if I interpreted your slide correctly, you had equal reaction with estrone and estradiol. Is that correct?

N. JIANG.   Yes.

W. ODELL.   Others have reported today considerably less cross-reaction of anti-estradiol for estrone. Thus, we have a good demonstration of the variation in specificity possible with antiserum directed against a single steroid conjugated in identical fashions. Even with steroids, it does not appear that we may direct antibody specificity with full reliability.

N. JIANG.   This morning Dr. Odell was interested in finding out if there are steroid antisera developed from other species besides rabbit and sheep. Some of you may want to try to produce antiserum from other species. If so, I have several guinea pigs which were immunized for 9 months. However, I did not get any antibody from them.

K. CATT.   Did you use any other type of tubes except those made of the one material that you mentioned, namely polystyrene? I ask this because, so far at this meeting, people have mainly mentioned the use of polystyrene, while in fact most plastics can be used successfully for this type of adsorption of antibody. The types of plastics we have found useful so far include polystyrene, which is the least expensive, polystyrene acrylonitrile, polyethylene, polypropylene, and also nylon.

S. TILLSON.   We have used only polystyrene tubes.

S. GROSS.   With regard to the specificity of antibodies directed against estradiol and estrone, I would like to ask, at what position was your steroid coupled to the protein carrier?

S. TILLSON.   Estradiol was coupled at the 17 position.

S. GROSS.   That is what I thought. I wonder if you would explain to me how the immune mechanism could be expected to recognize the difference between estradiol and estrone, when one is coupled at C-17. Sterically, the difference is minor.

G. ABRAHAM.   When we say we are blocking the hydroxyl by adding a succinate, in fact we are protecting that hydroxyl. We should not forget that having a succinate in the 17β position does not remove the hydrogen in the 17α position, whereas in estrone, there is no 17α hydrogen and the ketone group modifies the steric configuration of the ring bonds. There is also a different electronic structure. Antibodies are usually directed against the whole steroid, the succinate, and also against part of the lysine residue. For instance, one antibody preparation against estradiol-17β-hemisuccinate-BSA cross-reacted 120 percent with estradiol-17β-monoacetate, 150 percent with estradiol-17β-monopropionate, and 200 percent with estradiol-17β-monosuccinate. Estradiol-17β was 100 percent. The limit of the surface of the antibody active site has been estimated to be about 200 to 2,000Å square. The surface of the alpha side of the steroid, being about 60Å square, is even below the lower limit. Therefore, one would expect anti-estradiol-17β antibodies to be directed against not only the steroid, but the whole succinate, and even part of the lysine residue. I would expect antibodies to be able to differentiate between estrone and estradiol-17β even when a steroid-protein conjugate coupled at the 17β position is used for immunization. The succinate may prevent the biologic oxidation of estradiol-17β to estrone, making it a desirable feature.

8

HAPTEN-RADIOIMMUNOASSAY FOR STEROID HORMONES

Gordon D. Niswender and A. Rees Midgley, Jr.

The Reproduction and Endocrinology Program
Department of Pathology
The University of Michigan
Ann Arbor, Michigan

INTRODUCTION

One of the major advantages of using radioimmunoassay techniques for the measurement of steroid hormones is their unique potential for quantitating these hormones in unextracted serum, providing a truly specific antibody can be obtained to a given steroid. However, data regarding the factors which influence the specificity of antibodies to steroid hormones are incomplete. Since the basic structure of all steroid hormones is similar, i.e., they all contain the same basic cyclopentanophenanthrene nucleus, they offer an unequaled opportunity to study how minor alterations of this basic structure influence their immuno-reactivity. The structure of all steroid hormones differs only in the type and location of functional groups which are attached or introduced into this basic four ring nucleus.

In order to acquire a better understanding of what factors influence the specificity of antibodies produced against steroid hormones, a systematic approach was taken in the present studies to determine if differences in the specificity of antibodies to steroid hormones could be obtained by

This study was supported in part by a research grant (NIH-04105) and a contract (NIH-Contract-69-2134) from the National Institute of Child Health and Human Development and by a grant (369) from the Michigan Memorial Phoenix Project.

varying the position through which the steroid molecule was conjugated to protein.

Although tritiated steroids are used for quantitation in all of the existing methods for measuring steroids by competitive protein binding or radioimmunoassay techniques, there are potential advantages to the use of other radioisotopes for labeling steroid hormones for use in radioimmunoassays. If extraction and chromatographic purification of the sample are necessary, the procedural losses for individual samples should be determined. The use of tritiated steroid hormones of high specific activity for the radioactive hormone in the assay procedure makes it difficult also to use this hormone for determination of procedural losses. The extreme sensitivity of these assay methods also precludes the use of ^{14}C steroids for either quantitation or recovery of the hormone. It also seems apparent that the specific activity of the radioactive hormone is at least one of the factors which limits the sensitivity of any assay system. The potential for increasing the effective specific activity of a steroid hormone by conjugating it to protein and then radioiodinating that protein is theoretically many times greater than the levels which can be obtained using tritium. Several experiments were conducted in the latter portion of this study to compare results obtained with tritiated steroid hormones to those obtained with steroids conjugated to different types of substances capable of being radioiodinated.

METHODS

Preparation of Steroid Protein Conjugates

STEROID DERIVATIVES.   In general, three techniques were used to prepare steroid derivatives. When conjugation was desired at a position which contained a hydroxyl group, either a hemisuccinate or a chlorocarbonate derivative was prepared, while an (o-carboxymethyl) oxime derivative was prepared if conjugation was desired through a ketone group. The techniques used were essentially those described by Erlanger et al., 1967. Hemisuccinate derivatives were made at the 17 position of testosterone; at the 21 position of aldosterone, corticosterone, cortisone, and deoxycorticosterone; and at the 3 position of pregnenolone and estradiol-17β. A chlorocarbonate derivative was made at the 11 position of progesterone and the 17 positions of testosterone and estradiol-17β. An (o-carboxymethyl) oxime derivative was made at the 3 position of progesterone and testosterone, at the 20 position of progesterone, and at the 17 position of estrone. Details of the preparation and isolation of the oxime derivative of progesterone at the 3 position and of the hemisuccinate derivatives at the 3 position of estradiol-17β and the 21 position of aldosterone will be published elsewhere. Briefly, the oxime derivative of Δ^4-pregnene-20β-ol-3-one was oxidized at the 20 position to yield progesterone-3- (o-carboxymethyl) oxime. Mixtures of the 3, the 17, and the bis-hemisuccinates of estradiol-17β were prepared, and estradiol-3-hemisuccinate was isolated by thin-layer chromatography. When mild conditions using catalytic amounts of pyridine were used, the hemisuccinate of aldosterone was formed at the 21 position.

In order to be certain that the derivatives isolated had the intended chemical-physical structure, every steroid derivative used in this study had its properties characterized either by infrared spectroscopy, nuclear magnetic resonance, ultraviolet spectrophotometry, or combinations of these procedures.

CONJUGATION TO PROTEIN.   In all cases the hemisuccinate and oxime derivatives were linked via an amide bond to ε-amino groups in bovine serum albumin (BSA) and rabbit serum albumin (RSA) using a mixed anhydride reaction (Erlanger et al., 1967). In addition, several of the steroid derivatives were conjugated in a similar fashion to tyrosine methyl ester (TME) as described by Oliver et al., 1968. In the case of the chlorocarbonate derivatives a Schotten-Baumann reaction was used for conjugation of the steroid to protein. The ratio of the number of steroid molecules to protein molecules was determined by using trace levels of radioactive steroids in the starting material and determining the radioactivity present in a weighed portion of the conjugate, or by UV analyses as described by Erlanger et al., 1958. In most cases, both methods were carried out concurrently and good agreement was observed between the two methods.

Radioimmunoassay Procedures

IMMUNIZATION.   Six rabbits were immunized with three dose levels (two at 0.25 mg, two at 1.25 mg, and two at 6.25 mg) of each steroid-protein conjugate. The antigen was emulsified in complete Freund's adjuvant and administered into the footpads and multiple subcutaneous sites. Each rabbit was injected with the same dose level three times with 3-week intervals between injections. They were bled at weekly intervals beginning 2 weeks after the last injection.

The preparation of the anti-rabbit gamma globulin (RGG) used in these studies has been described by Niswender et al. (1969).

RADIOIODINATION.   The steroid hormones were conjugated to rabbit serum albumin (RSA) and to tyrosine methyl ester (TME) for radioiodination. RSA was used in the initial studies because of its high content of tyrosine residues and because it seemed unlikely that antiserum pro-

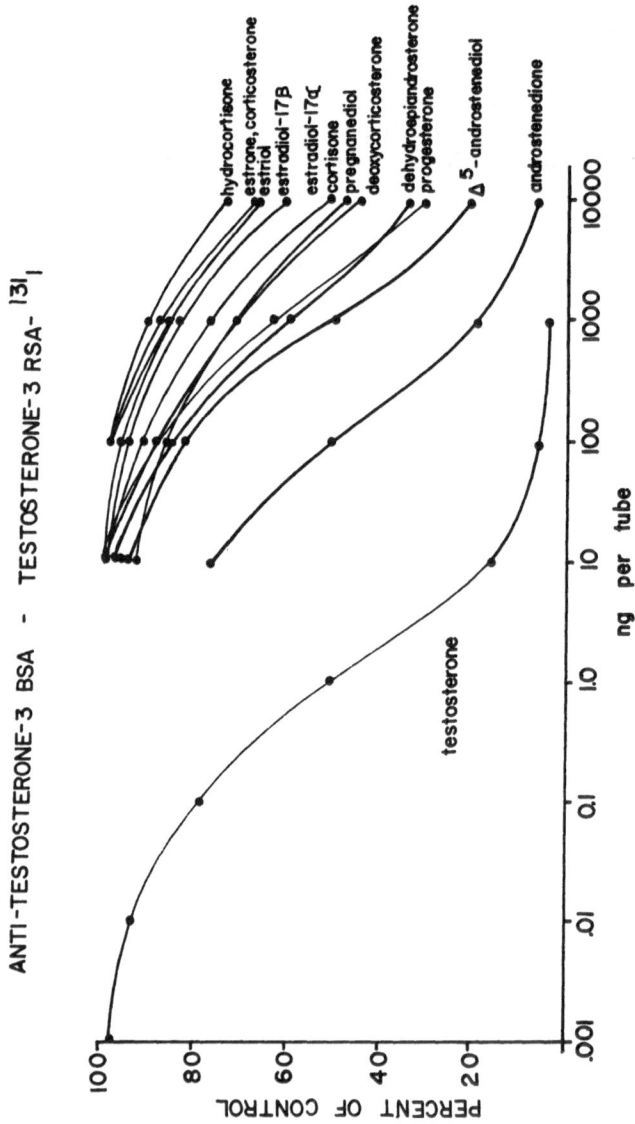

Fig. 1. Inhibition curves with selected steroids in the testosterone-3-RIA.

duced to BSA in rabbits would immunologically cross-react with RSA. To further insure that this possibility did not occur, all assays were done with 1 percent BSA in the buffer medium. Due to the relatively high number of steroid molecules (22 to 38 per RSA molecule) the steroid was also conjugated to TME to insure a ratio of one steroid per one protein molecule. Radioiodination was done by the method of Greenwood et al. (1963) as modified by Niswender et al. (1969).

RADIOIMMUNOASSAY.   The details of the double-antibody procedure used in these studies have been described by Niswender et al. (1969). In brief, this method consists of allowing 500 ml of combined sample or standard plus buffer to incubate with 200 µl of the appropriate dilution of antibody for 24 hours at 4°C, followed by the addition of 100 µl of radioactive hormone (steroid-RSA-^{131}I, steroid-TME-^{131}I, or steroid-^{3}H). After an additional 24 hours of incubation, 200 µl of anti-RGG were added and the incubation allowed to proceed for either 24 or 72 hours, depending upon whether unextracted serum was added to the assay tube (Midgley et al., 1969). The radioactivity in the precipitate from assay tubes which contained radioactive hormone and antibody, but which contained no unlabeled hormone (i.e., buffer control tubes), was assigned the value of 100 percent. As increasing amounts of unlabeled hormone were added the radioactivity bound to antibody was decreased in a dose-response manner (Fig. 1). All standard steroid preparations were purchased from Sigma Chemical Co. (St. Louis) and used as supplied. Due to the relative insolubility of many of the steroids in water, a concentrated solution (10 mg/ml) of all steroids used in these studies was made in dimethyl sulfoxide. Aliquots of these solutions were then diluted at least 1000-fold in the assay buffer so that appropriate steroid concentrations could be obtained.

RESULTS AND DISCUSSION

General

Data concerning the titer of antibody produced in rabbits to 11 different steroid antigens is shown in Table 1. The dilution of antibody referred to was the initial dilution used in the 200-µl aliquots, so the final dilution in each assay tube (1 ml) was five times greater than that shown. Steroid-RSA-^{131}I was used as the radioactive hormone and the percent bound reflects that proportion of the total radioactivity added which was bound to antibody in buffer control tubes. Significant antibody production occurred in all cases when approximately 20 or more steroid molecules were conjugated to each protein molecule. In fact, rea-

TABLE 1

Titer of Steroid Antibodies in Serum from Rabbits

Antigen	Steroid mol. Protein mol.	No. of rabbits	Reciprocal of dilution	Mean %[a] bound	Range % bound
Progesterone-11-BSA	36.0	6	1,200[b]	51.0	35-63
Progesterone-3-BSA	22.0	6	2,000	46.0	28-55
Pregnenolone-3-BSA	21.0	6	6,000	55.0	8-68
Estrone-17-BSA	28.0	6	6,000	32.0	12-49
Estradiol-3-BSA	18.0	6	2,000	68.0	63-72
Testosterone-3-BSA	28.0	6	6,000	35.0	17-55
Testosterone-17-BSA	22.0	6	6,000	67.0	57-81
Aldosterone-21-BSA	3.0	5	6,000	3.0	2-11
Corticosterone-21-BSA	7.8	6	6,000	3.0	2-33
Cortisone-21-BSA	7.0	6	6,000	16.0	6-34
Deoxycorticosterone-21-BSA	8.6	5	1,200	28.0	2-48

[a]Using steroid-RSA-^{131}I.
[b]The dilution of the bleeding two weeks after the third injection.

sonable titers of antibody were obtained in all but four of 42 rabbits immunized with seven different steroid antigens with 18 or more steroid molecules per protein molecule. However, when there were less than 10 steroid molecules per BSA molecule, as was the case with all corticosteroid conjugates, the titer of antibody was low or otherwise unsuitable for radioimmunoassay in 22 rabbits. Since others (Erlanger et al., 1958) have successfully produced antibodies to adrenal cortical hormones, we have concluded that we did not have sufficient numbers of steroid molecules conjugated to BSA to elicit suitable antibody production.

These data demonstrate that rabbits are suitable animals for the production of antibodies to steroid hormones and further suggest that a ratio of approximately 20 or more steroid molecules per protein molecule is efficacious for antibody production.

Testosterone Radioimmunoassay

Two radioimmunoassay (RIA) procedures were developed for testosterone, one using anti-testosterone-3-BSA serum and testosterone-3-RSA-^{131}I and the other using anti-testosterone-17-BSA serum and testosterone-17-RSA-^{131}I. Inhibition curves with 14 selected steroids in each of these systems are shown in Figures 1 and 2. In both assay systems the inhibition curves appear to be similar in shape and slope. In subsequent experiments, when most steroids were tested to the limits of their solubility in aqueous media, most steroids were capable of totally inhibiting the binding of testosterone-RSA-^{131}I to antibody. A numerical estimation of the relative activity of these selected steroid hormones in the two assay systems is shown in Table 2. The differences in the chem-

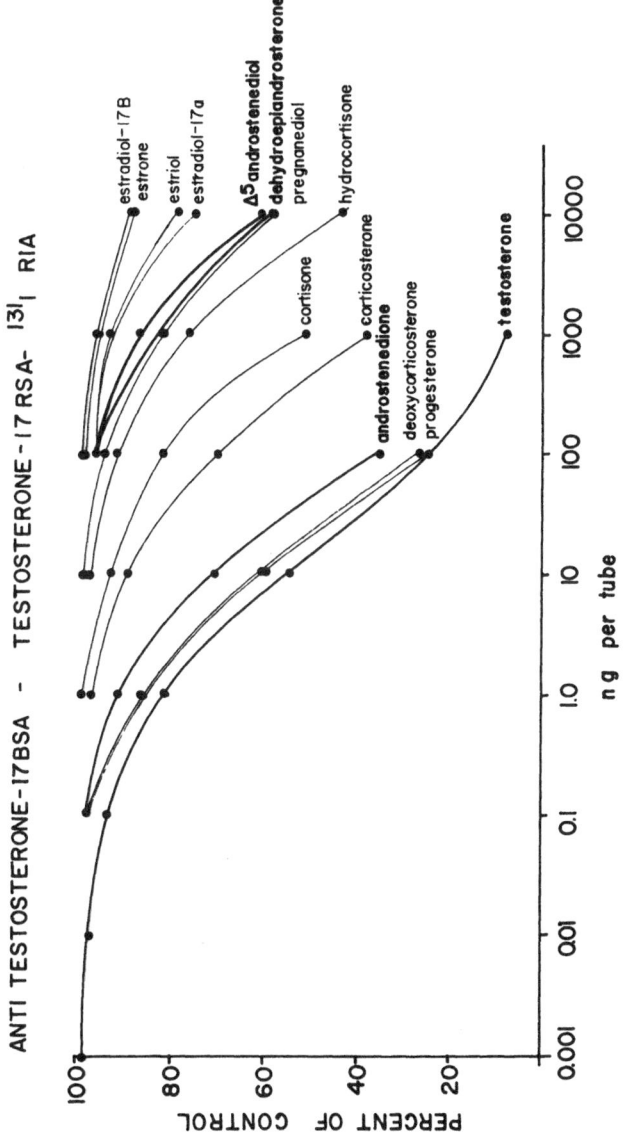

Fig. 2. Inhibition curves with selected steroids in the testosterone-17-RIA.

TABLE 2

Relative Activity[a] of Selected Steroids in Different Testosterone Radioimmunoassays

Steroid	Testosterone-3[b]	Testosterone-17[c]
Testosterone	1.00	1.00
Ardrostenediol	.013	.0005
Androstenedione	.002	.31
Deoxycorticosterone	.0018	.55
Dehydroepiandrosterone	.0005	.001
Estradiol-17β	.0004	<.0001
Progesterone	.0004	.55
Corticosterone	.0003	.029
Cortisone	.0001	.009
Estradiol-17α	<.0001	<.0001
Estriol	<.0001	<.0001
Pregnanediol	<.0001	.0008
Hydrocortisone	<.0001	.002
Pregnenolone	<.0001	<.0001

[a] Relative activity = $\dfrac{\text{ng of testosterone at 50\%}}{\text{ng of steroid x at 50\%}}$

[b] Anti-testosterone-3-BSA; testosterone-3-RSA-[131] I.

[c] Anti-testosterone-17-BSA; testosterone-17-BSA-[131] I.

ical structure of four of the androgenic steroid hormones and progesterone and estradiol-17β are illustrated in Figure 3. In the testosterone-3-RIA, any differences in the chemical structure of the steroid molecule which occurred at the end of the molecule away from the site of protein conjugation drastically reduced the relative activity of the steroid

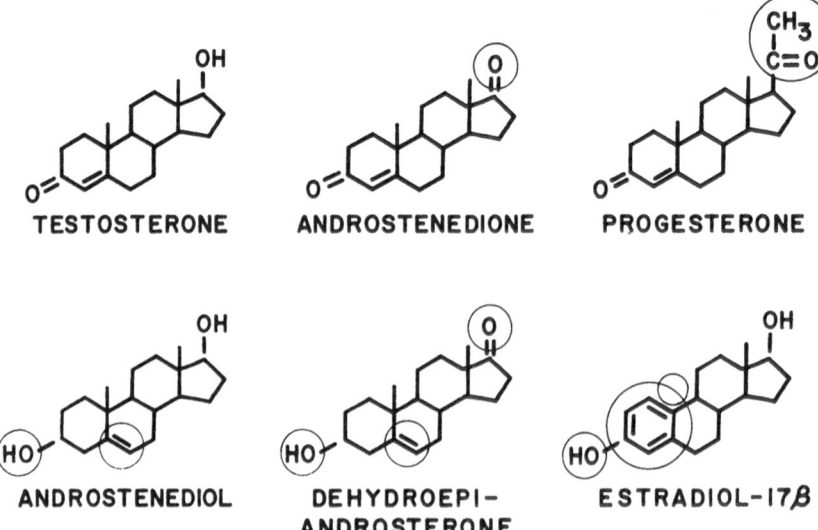

Fig. 3. Structural formulas for four androgenic steroid hormones and for progesterone and estradiol-17β. Circles indicate those portions of the molecule which differ in structure from that found in testosterone.

(i.e., androstenedione, progesterone, dehydroepiandrosterone). This same observation was true for the other steroids tested. In addition, alterations of the steroid molecule which occurred near the site of protein conjugation also reduced the relative activity of the steroid in the testosterone-3-RIA (i.e., androstenediol, estradiol-17β). It should be noted that the bond angles and the conformational structure of the steroid molecule are altered considerably when the 17-hydroxyl group is changed to a 17-ketone, or when the Δ^4-double bond-3-ketone configuration is changed to a Δ^5-double bond-3-hydroxyl as occurs in androstenediol and dehydroepiandrosterone. The structure of the phenolic A ring in estradiol-17β is planar compared to the coplanar A ring of testosterone. From these data it appears that antibodies to testosterone-3-BSA can distinguish differences in the testosterone molecule which occur at either end of the molecule. Since hormones which contain these alterations are capable of completely inhibiting the binding of testosterone-3-RSA-^{131}I to the antibody, with an inhibition curve parallel to that for testosterone (although testosterone is at least 80 times more reactive), it was concluded that the major portion of the entire steroid molecule is functioning as a single antigenic site.

In the testosterone-17-RIA, differences in the steroid molecule in the end opposite to where the protein had been conjugated (androstenediol, dehydroepiandrosterone, estradiol-17β) again drastically reduced the relative activity of these steroid hormones (Table 2). However, differences occurring near the site of protein conjugation had little effect on the activity of the molecule. The presence of a ketone group at the 17 position (androstenedione) or the presence of additional carbon atoms along with their reactive groups (progesterone, deoxycorticosterone) did little to alter the relative activity of these steroid hormones in the testosterone-17-RIA.

It was concluded from these data that a relatively specific antibody can be produced against testosterone if one conjugates this steroid to protein at the 3 position. The principal differences between the various 19-C and the 21-C steroids occur in the C and D rings of the molecule; therefore the protein should not be conjugated through the 17 position on the D ring if one wishes to obtain a specific antibody for testosterone. This portion of the molecule should be left available to incur specificity to the antibody.

Since these data suggested that the testosterone-3-RIA for testosterone was reasonably specific, we attempted to quantitate the levels of testosterone in unextracted serum. As can be seen in Table 3, the agreement between RIA and gas-liquid chromatography estimates was quite good for the testosterone content of several samples of serum from male rats. There was no detectable testosterone in serum from castrated, adrenalectomized rats by either method. The gas-chromatographic

TABLE 3

Serum Levels of Testosterone in Male Rats

Rat	G.C.[a] (ng/ml)	RIA (ng/ml)	G.C./RIA
Normal male	3.7	3.5	1.05
Normal male	2.1	1.9	1.10
Normal male	4.3	4.3	1.00
Normal male	2.8	2.4	1.16
Normal male	3.3	2.6	1.32
Pool from males	1.2	1.7	0.71
Pool from males	4.6	7.2	0.64
Castrate, adrenalectomized	N.D.[b]	N.D.	
Castrate, adrenalectomized	N.D.	N.D.	

[a]Data from Kirschner and Coffman, 1969.
[b]There was no detectable testosterone in these samples.

analyses were done by M. A. Kirschner as described by Kirschner and Coffman (1969). Good agreement was also obtained when a comparison was made between RIA and competitive protein binding (CPB) estimates for the testosterone in serum from male sheep. However, when unextracted serum samples from female rats or sheep were run in the testosterone-3-RIA, the values obtained were as much as 10 times higher than those obtained by CPB. The CPB analyses were done by R. Wieland as described by Hallberg et al. (1968). When serum samples from women were analyzed in the testosterone-3-RIA and the values compared to those obtained with a double-isotope derivative technique, the agreement between the two methods was poor, with the RIA method usually overestimating the testosterone content. The double-isotope derivative measurements were done by J. Lobotsky as described by Riondell et al. (1963).

It was concluded from these data that the testosterone-3-RIA was being influenced by some steroid (or steroids) which was present in substantial quantities in female blood and which was not one of the major steroids which had been tested in the assay, or that steroid-binding proteins present in blood from females were interfering in the assay. Studies are presently underway to determine if either of these possibilities is actually the cause of the overestimation of testosterone in serum from females.

Progesterone Radioimmunoassay

In an attempt to develop a specific antibody to progesterone, BSA was conjugated at the 3 and 20 positions. It was also possible to conjugate BSA to progesterone at the 11 position by using the chlorocarbonate derivative of 11-OH progesterone. Pregnenolone was also conjugated to BSA at the 3 position for immunization. The relative activity of 19 major steroids was tested in each of the four assay systems. Differences in

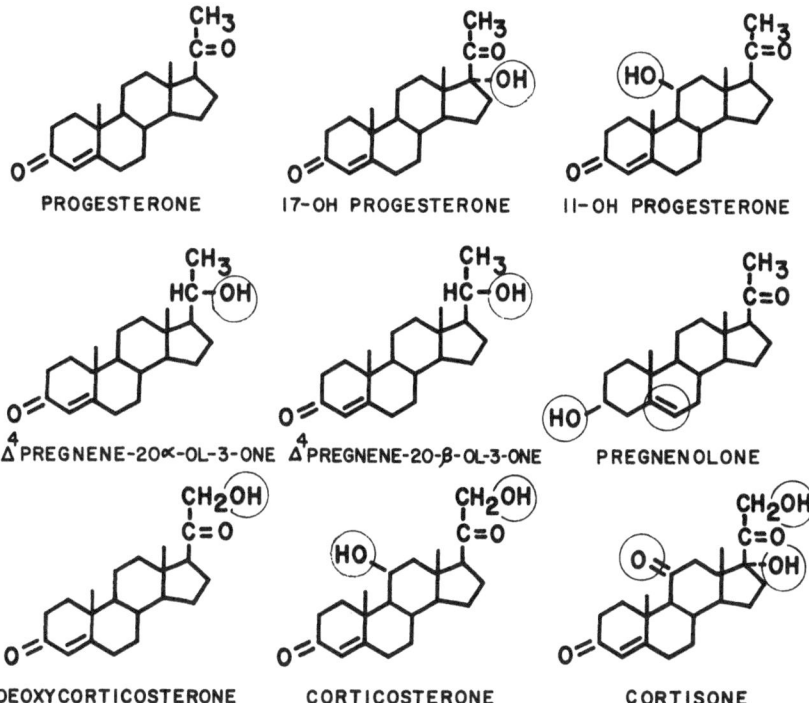

Fig. 4. Structural formulas for nine 21-C steroid hormones. Circles indicate those portions of the molecule which differ in structure from that found in progesterone.

the structure of nine selected C-21 steroids are illustrated in Figure 4. In the progesterone-3-RIA, C-21 steroids with hydroxyl groups at the 11, 17, 20α and 20β, or 21 positions had considerably reduced immunoreactivity when compared to progesterone. The 3-hydroxyl, Δ⁵-double bond configuration in pregnenolone also reduced its relative activity. The absence of C atoms at the 20 and 21 positions in testosterone also drastically reduced reactivity as did combinations of hydroxyl and ketone groups at the 11, 17, and 21 positions.

In the progesterone-20-RIA, steroids with differences in the structure of the A, B, or C rings were all considerably less reactive than progesterone. However, those steroids with structures identical to progesterone in the A, B, C, and D rings (Fig. 4) including 17-OH progesterone deoxy-corticosterone, Δ⁴-pregnene-20β-ol-3-one, and testosterone were essentially as immuno-reactive as progesterone. Δ⁴-pregnene-20α-ol-3-one had one-third the reactivity of progesterone (Table 4).

The progesterone-11-RIA was unique in that the protein was conjugated to the middle of the progesterone molecule, thus leaving both ends available to incur specificity to the antibody. Differences in the

TABLE 4

Relative Activity[a] of Selected Steroids in Different Progesterone Radioimmunoassays

Steroids	Proges-terone-3[b]	Proges-terone-20[c]	Proges-terone-11[d]	Pregnen-olone-3[e]
Progesterone	1.00	1.00	1.00	1.00
Pregnenolone	.13	.011	.005	1.70
11-OH-progesterone	.13	.071	.345	.133
17-OH-progesterone	.046	.981	.012	.060
Deoxycorticosterone	.016	.965	.007	.060
Corticosterone	.004	.004	.002	.007
Δ^4-pregnene-20β-ol-3-one	.003	.965	.001	.035
Δ^4-pregnene-20α-ol-3-one	.001	.336	.001	.039
Testosterone	.0005	.952	.0004	.003
Aldosterone	.0004	.071	.0001	.007
Cortisone	.0002	.056	.0003	.007
Hydrocortisone	.0002	.004	<.0001	.007
Cholesterol	.0001	.003	<.0001	.004
Pregnanediol	<.0001	.003	<.0001	<.0001
Estradiol-17α	<.0001	.0004	<.0001	<.0001
Estradiol-17β	<.0001	<.0001	<.0001	<.0001
Estrone	<.0001	<.0001	<.0001	<.0001
Estriol	<.0001	<.0001	<.0001	<.0001

[a] Relative activity = $\dfrac{\text{ng of progesterone at 50\%}}{\text{ng of steroid x at 50\%}}$

[b] Anti-progesterone-3-BSA; progesterone-3-TME-[131]I.

[c] Anti-progesterone-20-BSA; progesterone-20-TME-[131]I.

[d] Anti-progesterone-11-BSA; progesterone-11-RSA-[131]I.

[e] Anti-pregnenolone-3-BSA; pregnenolone-3-RSA-[131]I.

structure at either end of the steroid molecule considerably reduced the immuno-reactivity of the different steroids in this assay system. All of the steroids tested, except 11-OH progesterone, had less than 1 percent of the reactivity of progesterone in the progesterone-11-RIA.

It was concluded from these data that a fairly specific antibody to progesterone could be obtained by the conjugation of BSA at the 3 position, but an even more specific antibody was obtained when the protein was conjugated at the 11 position, leaving both ends of the progesterone molecule available to incur specificity to the antibody. Attempts to measure progesterone in unextracted serum in either the progesterone-3-RIA or the progesterone-11-RIA have been unsuccessful to date.

As a concluding experiment in this portion of the study, pregnenolone was conjugated to BSA and RSA at the 3 position. The specificity of the resulting RIA was similar to that noted in the progesterone-3-RIA. Differences in the steroid molecule which occurred in the C or D rings considerably reduced the immuno-reactivity of that steroid. The structural differences in the A and B rings of progesterone resulted in its being slightly less reactive than pregnenolone in the pregnenolone-3-RIA.

TABLE 5

Relative Activity[a] of Selected Steroids in Different Estrogen Radioimmunoassays

Steroid	Estradiol-3[b]	Estradiol-17[c]	Estrone-17[d]
Estradiol-17β	1.00	1.00	.04
Estradiol-17α	.30	.47	.018
Estrone	.67	.96	1.00
Estriol	.22	.10	.015
Testosterone	.0002	.0005	—
Progesterone	.0001	.0009	.0005
Deoxycorticosterone	.0001	.0001	.0005
Costicosterone	<.0001	.0002	.0005
Cortisone	<.0001	<.0001	.0001

[a] Relative activity = $\dfrac{\text{ng of estradiol-17 or estrone at 50\%}}{\text{ng of steroid x at 50\%}}$

[b] Anti-estradiol-3-BSA; estradiol-3-TME-[131] I.

[c] Anti-estradiol-17-BSA; estradiol-17-BSA-[131] I.

[d] Anti-estrone-17-BSA; estrone-17-RSA-[131] I.

Estrogen Radioimmunoassays

In order to study how the site of conjugation affects the specificity of antibodies to estradiol-17β, this steroid was conjugated to BSA at the 3 position or at the 17 position. Estrone was also conjugated to BSA at the 17 position. A comparison of the three resulting RIAs is shown in Table 5. In the estradiol-3-RIA all of the phenolic steroids possessed considerable immuno-reactivity. However, slight differences were noted when

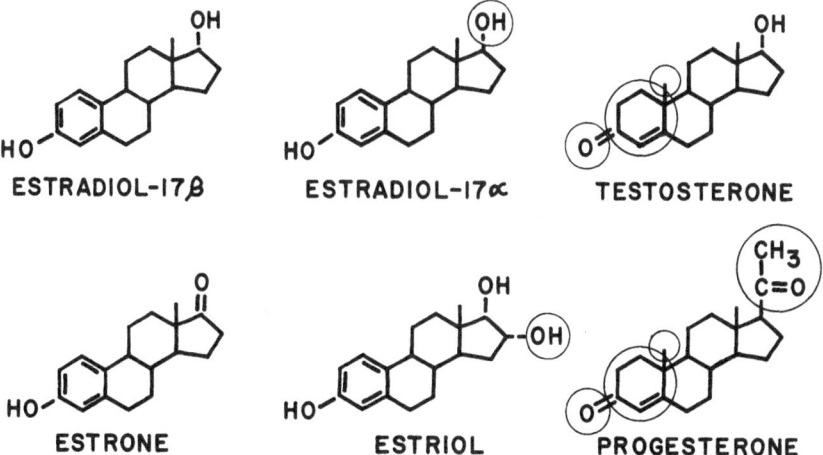

Fig. 5. Structural formulas for four phenolic steroid hormones and testosterone and progesterone. Circles indicate those portions of the molecule which differ in structure from that found in estradiol-17β or estrone.

a 17α-hydroxyl group, a 17-ketone, or a 16α-hydroxyl group was present (Fig. 5). All of the steroids tested which did not contain a phenolic A ring were at least 5000 times less reactive in this system than estradiol-17β.

A result similar to that noted in the estradiol-3-RIA was obtained in the estradiol-17-RIA. All of the phenolic steroids possessed considerable immuno-reactivity although there were slight differences between them. Again the absence of a phenolic A ring reduced the reactivity of the steroid at least 10,000 times when compared to estradiol-17β.

In the estrone-17-RIA the presence of a 17α-OH, a 17β-OH, or the combination of a 17β-OH and a 16α-OH in the 18-C steroids all greatly reduced immuno-reactivity. Again, as in the estradiol-3-RIA and the estradiol-17-RIA all of the steroids tested in the estrone 17-RIA which did not contain a phenolic A ring had very low immuno-reactivity.

It was concluded from these studies that antibodies which were quite capable of distinguishing phenolic steroids from neutral steroids could be produced with estradiol conjugated to BSA at either the 3 or 17 positions. However, at least with a limited number of rabbits we were not able to produce an antibody to estradiol which clearly differentiated between the four phenolic steroids. On the other hand, a reasonably specific antibody was obtained to estrone-17-BSA, and in the RIA system which used this antibody the other phenolic steroids were less than 4 percent as reactive as estrone. No attempt has been made to quantitate either estradiol-17β or estrone in unextracted serum.

In a final series of experiments we attempted to compare several forms of radioactive steroid for use in the radioimmunoassay. Inhibition curves were obtained with all forms of radioactive hormone tested in the estrone-17-RIA (Fig. 6) including estrone-^{3}H, estrone 17-RSA-^{131}I, estrone TME-^{131}I and estrone TME-[125]I. In each case the antibody was appropriately diluted so that approximately 45 percent of the total radioactivity was bound to antibody in buffer control tubes. The assay was more sensitive and precise when estrone-TME was used for radioiodination due to the slope of the inhibition curve.

It should be pointed out that there was a 5- to 10-fold difference in count rate between the radioiodinated preparations and the high-specific-activity estrone-^{3}H used in this study. This implies that each assay tube would have to be counted at least five times longer to achieve the same level of counting statistics when estrone-^{3}H was used. In addition, if radioiodinated forms of the steroid are used in the RIA, the tritiated steroid can be reserved for the determination of procedural losses if extraction and chromatography are necessary.

A similar comparison of estradiol-3-TME-^{131}I and estradiol-^{3}H is shown in Figure 7. It should be pointed out that in this assay system as little as 10 pg of estradiol per assay tube can be reliably quantitated. Inhibition curves using progesterone-^{3}H and progesterone-TME-^{131}I are

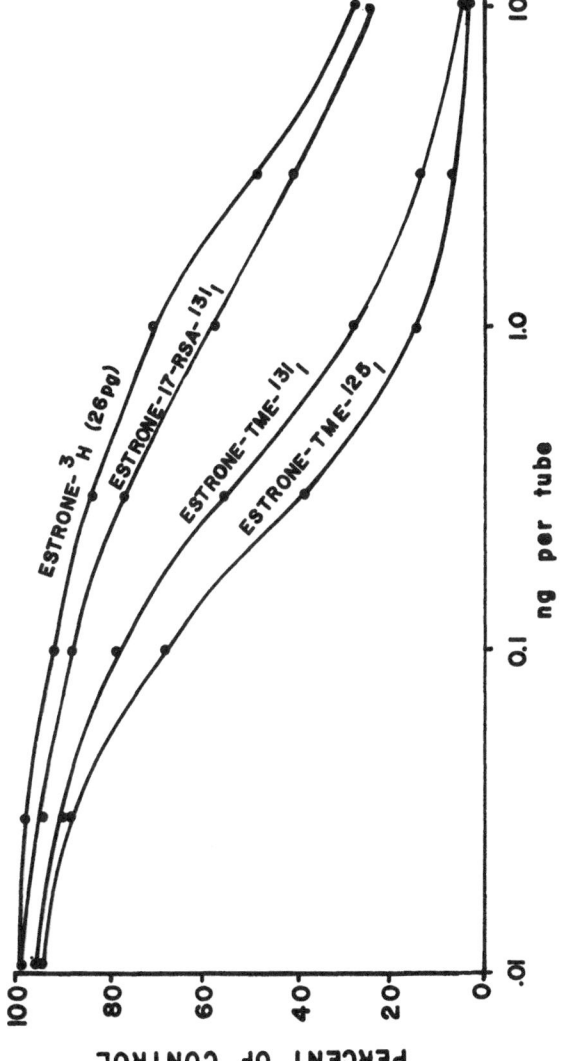

Fig. 6. Inhibition curves with different forms of radioactive estrone in the estrone-17-RIA.

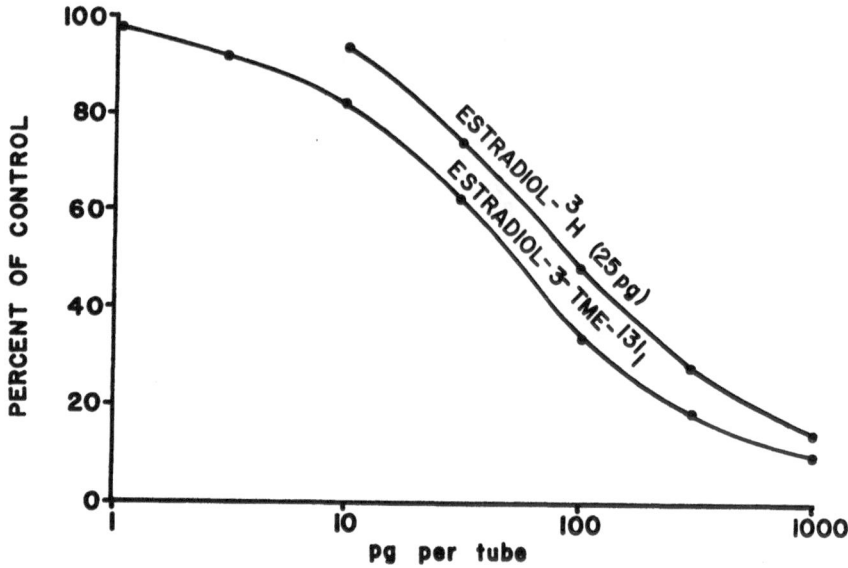

Fig. 7. Inhibition curves with high specific activity estradiol-17β-³H and estradiol-3-TME-¹³¹I in the estradiol-3-RIA.

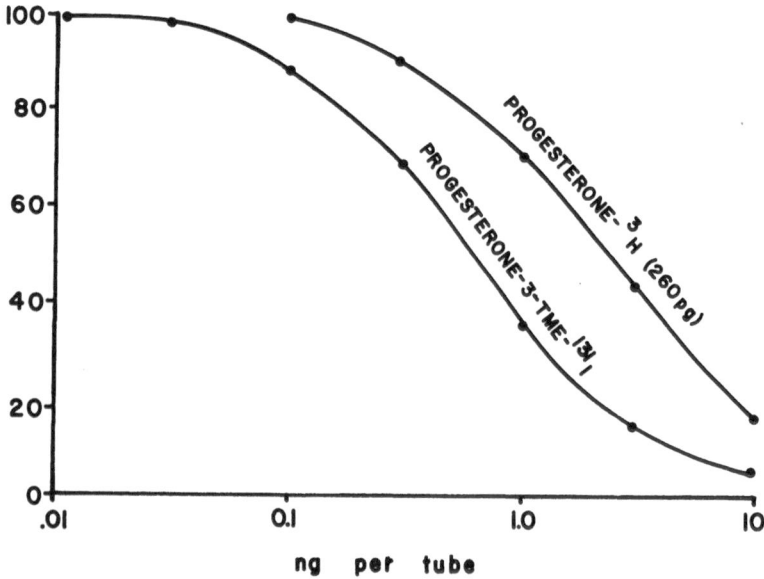

Fig. 8. Inhibition curves with progesterone-³H and progesterone-3-TME-¹³¹I in the progesterone-3-RIA.

shown in Figure 8. It was concluded from these experiments that radioiodination of steroid protein conjugates was a suitable method for obtaining radioactive steroids for use in radioimmunoassays.

SUMMARY

It was determined from these experiments that high-titered, reasonably specific antibodies to steroid hormones could be produced consistently in rabbits immunized with steroid-BSA conjugates if approximately 18 or more steroid molecules were present on each BSA molecule. In general, it appeared that to develop specific antibodies to neutral steroid hormones it was desirable to conjugate the BSA through the 3 position, since most of the differences in the various neutral steroids occur in the functional groups attached to the C or D rings. For progesterone it may be even better to conjugate BSA at the 11 position, leaving both ends of the molecule available to incur specificity to the antibody. These data might also suggest that more specific antibodies could be obtained if other steroids were conjugated to BSA at a position in the B or C rings. Although an RIA was developed which appeared to be specific for the measurement of testosterone in unextracted serum from males, the assay consistently overestimated the testosterone content of unextracted serum from female rats, sheep, or humans. Antibodies produced against phenolic steroid hormones cross-reacted only slightly with neutral steroid hormones, but all of the estrogens cross-reacted considerably with antibodies produced with estradiol-3- or estradiol-17-BSA. However, estradiol-17β, estradiol-17α, and estriol were all at least 20 times less reactive than estrone in an estrone-17-RIA.

In addition, data obtained in a portion of these studies demonstrated that radioiodinated steroid-protein conjugates could be used as the radioactive form of these hormones in radioimmunoassays. Inhibition curves obtained with steroid-TME-^{131}I were more sensitive than those obtained with steroid-[3]H. The higher specific activity associated with this radioiodinated form of steroid hormones made it possible to obtain reliable counting statistics in considerably less time and with less expense. Tritiated steroids can be used to determine recoveries of individual samples if radioiodinated steroids are used in the radioimmunoassays.

Acknowledgments

The authors wish to acknowledge the provision of serum samples with known testosterone contents by Dr. C. Lloyd and Julia Lobotsky of the Worcester Foundation for Experimental Biology, by Dr. W. Bardin of the Endocrine Section, National Institutes of Health, and by Dr. R. G. Wieland of Case Western Reserve University.

The technical assistance of Mr. J. Hudson and Mrs. M. Hepburn is gratefully acknowledged.

REFERENCES

Erlanger, B. F., F. Borek, S. M. Beiser, and S. Lieberman. 1958. Preparation and characterization of conjugates of bovine serum albumin with testosterone and with cortisone. J. Biol. Chem., 228:713, 727.

—— S. M. Beiser, F. Borek, F. Edel, and S. Lieberman. 1967. *In* Williams, C. A. and M. C. Chase, eds. Methods in Immunology and Immuno Chemistry. New York, Academic Press, Inc. Vol. 1, pp. 144, 151.

Greenwood, F. C., W. M. Hunter, and J. S. Glover. 1963. The preparation of ^{131}I-labelled human growth hormone of high specific activity. Biochem. J., 89:114–123.

Hallberg, M. C., E. M. Zorn, and R. G. Wieland. 1968. A sensitive testosterone assay by protein-binding. Steroids, 12:241, 248.

Kirschner, M. A., and G. D. Coffman. 1969. Measurement of plasma testosterone and Δ^4-androstenedione using electron capture gas-liquid chromatography. J. Clin. Endocr., 28:1347, 1355.

Midgley, A. R., R. W. Rebar, and G. D. Niswender. 1969. Radioimmunoassays employing double-antibody techniques. *In* Diczfalusy, E, Proc. 1st Karolinska Symposium: Immunoassay of Gonadotrophins. p. 163.

Niswender, G. D., L. E. Reichert, A. R. Midgley, and A. V. Nalbandov. 1969. Radioimmunoassay for bovine and ovine luteinizing hormone. Endocrinology, 84:1166–1173.

Oliver, G. C., B. M. Parker, D. L. Brasfield, and C. W. Parker. 1968. The measurement of digitoxin in human serum by radioimmunoassay. J. Clin. Invest., 47:1035, 1042.

Riondel, A., J. F. Tait, M. Gut, S. A. S. Tait, E. Joachim, and B. Little. 1963. Estimation of testosterone in human peripheral blood using S^{35}-thiosemicarbazide. J. Clin. Endocr., 23:620, 628.

DISCUSSION

S. Gross. How many milligrams of immunoglobulin G did you bring down with your second antibody, and how much antibody was left in solution? If this is unknown the supernatant may retain a considerable amount of soluble antibody-steroid complex. While your data demonstrated a degree of specificity for polar groups, a large number of antibodies are directed to the steroid backbone. Although the aromatic A ring is highly important there is no question that C-3 plays a role in specificity as well. Perhaps, as in enzyme kinetics, both positions C-3 and C-17 interact. It is reasonable to postulate that the C-17 imparts specificity and C-3 contributes to stabilization of the interaction. Your inhibition data are interesting. If it is possible to block an antibody with a variety of steroids, the population you detect may be primarily those directed against the backbone. It would seem obvious that we need to detect differences in related steroids if an assay is to have clinical application.

G. NISWENDER. The intent of these studies was to develop specific radioimmunoassays; therefore, the particular antibodies which were useful for this purpose were the only ones which were studied. However, I think that if there were antibodies present in these antisera which were reacting with specific entities on the steroid molecule one would expect to demonstrate these antibodies in the test systems used. For example, if we had a portion of the antibodies in our T-3-RIA which were directed against the hydroxyl group at the 17 position, then it does not seem possible that either androstenedione or dehydroepiandrosterone could totally inhibit the binding of labeled testosterone to the antibody in a dose-response curve which was parallel to testosterone (Fig. 2). These substances should not be able to prevent the binding of labeled testosterone to those antibodies (if present) which were specific for the hydroxyl group at the 17 position, and therefore one would not expect the curve to go smoothly to 0 percent bound.

P. ZIMMERING. In earlier studies, we made antibodies to testosterone conjugated in both the 3 and 17 positions to study their binding. We found two very different kinds of binding sites—tight and loose sites. It is possible that you are not picking up the loose binding. We were concerned with the heterogeneity of the antibody-binding sites and applied the Sips equation to our binding studies. This equation contains an index of the heterogeneity of the binding affinities. We used a number of derivatives of testosterone with hydroxyl groups added at various positions and found that, as we got lower binding constants, we also got less heterogeneity. It may be that, in this whole population of binding sites, there are some steroid derivatives that will bind only to one of them with homogeneous binding for that hapten. But these are very loose sites. The fact that your system picks up only the tight binding makes it more useful for the present purpose.

G. NISWENDER. It certainly is possible that there is a very loose, low affinity type of binding which we are not detecting. I would also like to point out at this time that the response of each individual animal to a given antigen is unique, whether they be different rabbits or different sheep. Each individual produces antiserum with its own unique properties. However, when we tested the specificity of the antisera from four rabbits immunized with testosterone-3-BSA, we found that there were slight differences in the mathematical figures for reactivity with different steroids, but the general pattern was the same in every rabbit.

R. HORTON. Many of us are now evaluating our experience with the whole area of binding techniques, tissue proteins, and plasma proteins in the light of the new steroid antibodies as to the best approach. It would seem to me that, unless and until we have antibodies so specific that analysis can be made on unpurified biologic material, these other techniques are still quite competitive. The presence of relative nonspecificity for some of these antibodies would seem to be, in certain cases, an advantage as long as adequate purification, usually chromatography, is going to be used. The example might be given for other binding techniques—the use of cortisol-binding protein which has been successfully used for a host of steroids.

G. Niswender.   You are right. Obviously we are idealists and had hoped we could produce specific antibodies to allow us to measure steroids without extraction. This particular aspect has not been fruitful at the present time. However, we still feel that it is possible to develop specific assays and are pursuing this goal concurrently with the development of extraction and purification techniques.

B. Africa.   You stated you had haptens specifically bound at C-20 or C-3. How did you selectively react only with the one and not the other?

G. Niswender.   For conjugation at the 20 position we started with pregnenolone and used the methods described by Erlanger et al. (1967). We made the (o-carboxymethyl) oxime of progesterone at the 3 position of Δ^4-pregnene-20β-ol-3-one and then selectively oxidized at the 20 position to obtain a derivative of progesterone for conjugation at the 3 position.

A. R. Midgley.   I think, Dr. Horton, that it is now possible to almost custom design a binding protein to do whatever one wishes. It was not possible to do this in our initial studies, but as they have developed, we have predicted the type of immunologic cross-reactivities we will find. I think if a simple separation system exists for separation of two major classes of steroids, one could design a system to measure a specific steroid. If one wishes a nonspecific antiserum against all of the estrogens one can make this. I think these are great advantages of using antibodies. The association between the steroid and antibody will, I think, be considerably greater than that with the naturally occurring binding protein; and when one really designs an assay system that maximally utilizes that affinity, one will get a more sensitive radioimmunoassay than those reported here today.

S. Gross.   I must agree with Dr. Midgley. With physico-chemical measurements which are even easier to perform than radioimmunoassay, nonspecific binding of steroids to serum proteins does not represent a major problem. Several proteins may contribute. Binding to these and to inert IgG is weaker than to specific IgG. Allowances are made for this in calculating association constants by the Sips distribution.

W. Odell.   When you compared affinity for antibody binding sites for iodinated steroid conjugates and tritiated steroids, the mass of the two obviously must have been very different. Could you give us the information comparing on an equal mass basis, the reactivity of iodinated, ^{14}C, ^{3}H, and unlabeled steroid for any of the immunoassays you studied?

G. NISWENDER.   We have not done specific activity calculations on the RSA-^{131}I or the TME-^{131}I preparations. The problem for the RSA has been that we have no estimate of what proportion of the steroid molecules conjugated to protein is available to bind to the antibody. The actual mass of steroid added to each tube when conjugated to RSA was approximately the same as when tritiated steroid was used. Due to the small size of the steroid-TME conjugates, we cannot separate the radioiodinated form of these conjugates from free ^{131}I using biogel columns. We have had to use polyacrylamide gel disc electrophoresis and we have not devised a system for calculating specific activities with this technique at the present time, although it is certainly possible.

I. THORNEYCROFT.   I note one difference in your immunization procedures. In searching the literature, either intravenous or subcutaneous immunizations have been used. You used specifically the foot pad and seem to have had considerably more luck than most people in this field. I am wondering if you have also tried subcutaneous or intravenous injections and have had less success than with the foot pad?

G. NISWENDER.   We have not tried immunization schemes other than the one described. This method has been used in our laboratory for the glycoprotein hormones, and when initial immunizations with steroid-protein conjugates were successful we adopted the same procedure for steroid antigens. One is always hesitant to alter methods which have been very successful. For the same reasons we have not attempted to immunize other species.

L. AXELROD.   If indeed what we have heard this afternoon is true, and I believe it is, and we are permitted some speculation, should we not try to produce antibodies to estrogens using derivatives of estrogens? Perhaps if one really wants specificity one would make a 6β-hydroxyestradiol and then couple it to the protein like a lollypop. Then it has the entire molecule to skim for specificity. We can further speculate into the use of antiestrogens or antiandrogens in the case of certain cancers in which, instead of trying to surgically remove the carcinoma, we might cause regression of the tumors with antiestrogens or antiandrogens.

G. NISWENDER.   We certainly agree and feel quite strongly that it is optimal to make your conjugates at positions on the B and C rings which leaves both ends of the molecule available to incur specificity to the antibody.

A. WILHELMI.   Dr. Axelrod, I was thinking that just at the time when the steroid chemists had about exhausted all of the combinations and permutations, this technique now gives you an entirely new field in which to play. Isn't that gratifying!

A. R. MIDGLEY. Along these same lines it is fun to play with the possibilities, but it would seem to me that a really sharp physical protein chemist ought to be able to synthesize a substance which would fit very tightly to the region to which he wishes to bind. Rather than rely upon naturally synthesized antibodies one ought to build and make very specific binding substances. Is this impossible?

A. E. WILHELMI. Not impossible but it is improbable.

N. JIANG. I think as far as specificity is concerned I have a notion that maybe it is the time for us to begin to study the identities of all the interfering substances in the serum. I have some evidence that if you extract a serum exhaustively with ether as it is, eventually an ether extract can result which will not react in the immunoassay that we are using.

G. NISWENDER. We have not been successful in determining the identity of the substances which are interfering in our assays. If we adsorb serum obtained from males with charcoal, we can obtain serum which has absolutely no effect in our T-3-RIA. However, similar treatment of serum from females has no significant effect, suggesting that at least a portion of the substances from female serum which interfere in the testosterone assay are macromolecular.

C. MIGEON. I would like to report on our experience with the immunoassay of aldosterone in human plasma. Our work was started because of our frustration with the double-isotope dilution techniques. The investigation that I shall report here is actually the result of the efforts of Drs. Francis Bayard, Inese Beitins, and Avinoam Kowarski in my laboratory at The Pediatric Endocrine Clinic of The Johns Hopkins Hospital.

The preparation of the antigen was as follows: Pure crystalline aldosterone was acetylated with pyridine and acetic anhydride to the diacetate. The reason for this first step was an attempt to protect that part of the molecule that might give specificity to the antibody. The second step was the preparation of aldosterone-3-carboxymethoxime-18, 21-diacetate, using carboxymethoxyyamine hydrochloride and sodium acetate, in methanol, for 18 hours, at $25°C$. Then the derivative was coupled with rabbit albumin by the carbodiimide process.

An assay was carried out as shown in Procedure 1. In most of the work to be described, the rabbit plasma containing the antibody was diluted 1:100. Following a short incubation at $37°C$, a known amount of florisil was added to each test tube and, after shaking vigorously at $0°C$ for 20 minutes, an aliquot of the liquid phase was used for radioactivity counting in order to determine the percentage of the steroid which was bound to the antibody.

Procedure 1

The Assay

1 ml of 1% antibody preparation
+ 1,2-^{3}H-aldosterone
+ either known amount of aldosterone
   or unknown extract

     Shake at 37°C for 20 min (rotary evapo-mix)
     ice bath 0° for 10 min
     then add 30 mg florisil
     shake at 0°C for 20 min
     allow to stand in ice bath for 10 min

Adding known amounts of nonradioactive aldosterone to the assay, it was possible to obtain the standard curve shown in Figure 1. With a dilution of the antibody of 1:100, 100 pg of aldosterone can easily be differentiated from 0, and the curve obtained allowed for a fairly accurate measurement of up to 1,500 pg.

Studies of the specificity of the antibody are shown in Table I. If aldosterone is taken as 100 percent reference, then the percentage cross-reaction for cortisol was 0.005. Very little cross-reaction was observed

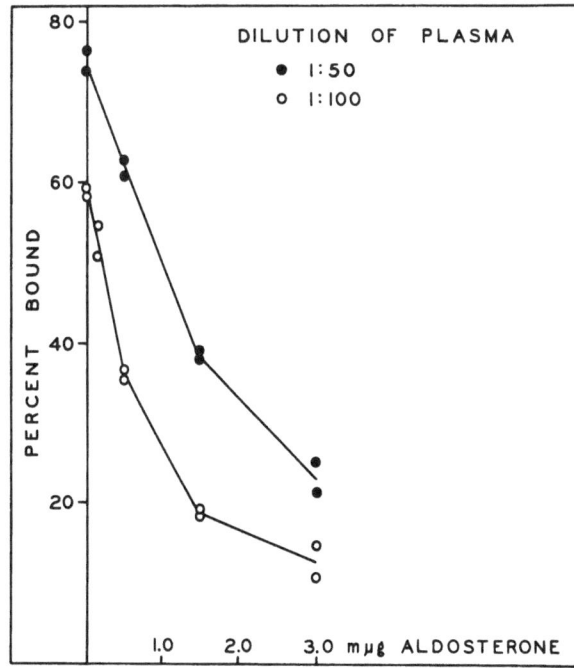

TABLE 1

Specificity of Antibody

Steroids		Percentage cross-reaction
21-C-steroids:	aldosterone	100.0
	cortisol	0.005
	cortisone	0.02
	11-desoxycortisol	0.004
	corticosterone	2.0
19-C-steroids:	testosterone	0.1
	androstenedione	0.1
18-C-steroids:	estradiol-17β	0.004
	estrone	0.004
	estriol	0.001

for either cortisone or 11-desoxycortisol. On the other hand, corticosterone had a 2 percent cross-reaction. Dr. Tait was kind enough to give us a small amount of nonradioactive 18-hydroxycorticosterone. Interestingly enough, this compound had a cross-reaction which was much less than that of corticosterone and which was somewhat similar to that of cortisol. A slight percentage of cross-reaction was found with androgens and a minimal one with estrogenic steroids.

At no time did we ever consider that we could work directly with plasma for the measurement of aldosterone. We therefore attempted to devise a fairly simple method for the preparation of a plasma extract. A tentative scheme is shown in Procedure 2. A small amount of 1, 2-^{3}H-aldosterone is added to 5 to 20 ml of plasma. Following extraction and one paper chromatography, an aliquot of the eluate is used for estimation of losses, while two other aliquots are used for a duplicate assay.

Procedure 2

Preparation of Plasma Extract

1. 5 to 20 ml plasma
   + 400 cpm 1,2-^{3}H-aldosterone
   + 0.4 ml 1.25 N NaOH

2. extraction with 15 volumes of cold CH_2Cl_2
   washing with 20 ml 0.1 N acetic acid once
   and 20 ml distilled water twice

3. evaporation of CH_2Cl_2 extract
   paper chromatography-benzene:methanol:water
   (100:50:50)

4. eluate divided in 3 equal aliquots
   one for recovery determination
   two for duplicate assay

Although we are still at the early stages of the development of the assay, and while further improvements are considered, it is possible to state presently that plasma aldosterone can be measured as described above. Reproducibility of results is good and specificity is not a problem if aldosterone is reasonably well separated from cortisol and cortisone.

It must be noted that several questions remained unanswered and several problems unresolved.

1. Nature of the antibody: It was our purpose to prepare the 3-carboxymethoxime of aldosterone-18, 21-diacetate. However, under the conditions used, the 18-acetate could have been hydrolyzed, and therefore a carboxymethoxime could have occurred also in this position. A third possibility would be reaction at the level of the 20-ketone; this is somewhat remote as one would expect that the 21-acetate group would render the 20-ketone inaccessible.

2. Titer of the antibody: The titer is rather low and it is necessary to use dilutions of rabbit plasma of 1:100 to 1:200. It might be that the titers will go up with further immunization. However, it must be emphasized that our present titer can permit an assay of aldosterone in human plasma.

3. Specificity: Specificity is very good. However, one must remember that the concentrations of aldosterone in plasma are low, varying between 2 and 20 ng/100 ml under conditions of normal sodium diet, while the normal concentrations of cortisol are 5 to 15 μg/100 ml. Since the study of cross-reaction shows that 20 μg of cortisol would equal 1 ng of aldosterone, it is quite apparent that cortisol must be carefully removed from plasma extracts prepared for aldosterone assay.

4. Blanks: Water blanks have been very low and in most cases of no significance.

5. Tritiated aldosterone added to the assay mixture for the construction of the standard curve: The small amount of 1, 2-^{3}H-aldosterone added to the assay mixture is about 50 pg and therefore the values on the abscissa of Figure 1 should all be increased by 50 pg. Recently, the use of radioactive aldosterone with two times the specific activity has decreased this amount to 25 pg.

9

THE USE OF AFFINITY CHROMATOGRAPHY IN THE PURIFICATION OF STEROID-BINDING PROTEINS

Sumner H. Burstein

Worcester Foundation for Experimental Biology
Shrewsbury, Massachusetts

INTRODUCTION

The term affinity chromatography seems to have been first used by Cuatrecasas et al. (1968); however, the principles involved have long been known in the field of immunology. In fact, as early as 1936, Landsteiner and van der Scheer used insolubilized haptens for the isolation of the corresponding antibodies. Since then numerous examples of antibody purification by use of immunosorbents have been reported (Silman and Katchalski, 1966).

The prodecure makes use of the specific affinity of the protein to be isolated for a second substance. In the case of an antibody, it would be the corresponding hapten; for an enzyme it would be either the substrate or an inhibitor. The substance is insolubilized, preferably by covalent linking to a suitable polymer, and the serum or other protein mixture allowed to interact with the adsorbent. If the system has been properly designed, only the desired protein will be removed from solution. After separation from the remaining components, the specifically adsorbed protein is eluted.

Several applications of this method to the isolation of steroid-binding proteins have been reported by others. Jensen et al. (1967) have described the separation of an estrogen receptor protein from calf uterine extract. The phenolic ring of estradiol was linked to *p*-aminobenzylcellulose by coupling of the diazonium derivative and the extract passed through a column of this adsorbent. Elution with desoxycholate yielded several milligrams of protein which exhibited some of the properties expected for the receptor. A similar study has been recently reported by Vonderhaar and Mueller (1969) who in addition prepared an estradiol adsorbent linked at 17α to a synthetic polymer. Using rat uterine preparations they were able to selectively and efficiently remove the estradiol-binding activity from solution. However, they had difficulty in eluting the protein in an active form due to its strong affinity for the adsorbent.

An anti-estrogen antibody has also been purified by means of an immunosorbent (Bauminger et al., 1969). Antiserum to the phyto-estrogen genistein was treated with an adsorbent consisting of a genistein derivative linked to cellulose. The antibody was successfully eluted with dilute acetic acid and used for a series of immunologic studies.

Some of the properties of testosterone-binding globulin (TeBG), which are necessary for the rational design of a specific adsorbent, have been studied (Vermeulen and Verdonck, 1968; Murphy, 1968; Heyns et al., 1969). In particular, the structural features of the steroid required for good binding are known. A 17β-hydroxyl group seems to be essential since the corresponding 17α-epimers or 17-keto steroids all bind weakly. The addition of an oxygen function at the 16 position also reduces binding markedly. In the A ring more variation in structure is possible without the loss of binding activity relative to testosterone. In fact, reduction of the double bond to a 5α configuration may lead to an increase in activity. Also the keto group at 3 can be replaced by either 3β- or 3α-hydroxyl with retention of binding.

The value of the binding constant is of obvious importance in considering a separation scheme of this type. In particular, it should be at least several orders of magnitude higher than that of any nonspecific binding proteins such as albumin which may be present. The published values (Vermeulen and Verdonck, 1968) for the equilibrium between TeBG and testosterone are around 10^8 liters/mole whereas albumin has a value of about 10^4 liters/mole. On the basis of this difference, the albumin trapped by a specific adsorbent should be displaced by TeBG.

After considering the above data and since there are convenient methods for insolubilizing amino-containing haptens, the steroid chosen for the adsorbent was 3β-aminoandrostan-17β-ol. Because the linkage to the polymer would be via the 3 position, the more essential D ring portion would be easily available for binding. The 5α stereochemistry is a favorable factor and, in addition, this compound was available commercially.

A general method for linking primary amines to polysaccharides has been developed which involves the use of cyanogen bromide as the coupling agent (Axen et al., 1967; Porath et al., 1967). The exact nature of the coupling reaction is not known; however, a stable covalent linkage is produced under relatively mild conditions. Both dextran and agarose preparations have been successfully used in making adsorbents with good physical as well as chemical properties. Agarose was chosen for this problem since it has a more open polymeric structure. Because of the small size of the hapten, easy access for the TeBG would be desirable for interaction between the active sites of the protein and the adsorbent.

TESTOSTERONE-BINDING GLOBULIN SEPARATION

The steroid was reacted with a cyanogen-bromide-agarose mixture in the ratio of about 3μEq. of steroid per gram of polymer. The completeness of the reaction was evidenced by the lack of free steroid after reaction even upon exhaustive solvent extraction of the complex. The physical characteristics of the agarose were unaltered by the steroid and freely flowing columns could be made.

The protein source was pooled human plasma which had been stored for 4 to 12 weeks at 4°C under sterile conditions. This was assayed for binding activity by equilibration with tritiated testosterone followed by separation of the bound and free hormone by gel filtration as described by Vermeulen and Verdonck (1968). By using a column of exact-specifications, a complete separation can be achieved without dissociation of the TeBG-testosterone complex. On the other hand, albumin-bound testosterone is completely dissociated, giving only the globulin binding in the protein peak.

A column containing about 2 g of the specific adsorbent was treated with 50 ml of undiluted plasma. The amount of steroid on the agarose was therefore about 10,000 times that of the testosterone in the plasma. The treated plasma was assayed for binding activity by the gel filtration technique and the results are shown in Table 1.

TABLE 1
Purification of Testosterone-Binding Globulin (TeBG)
by Affinity Chromatography of Pooled Human Plasma

	Testosterone bound[a] to protein[b] (dpm)	Protein concentration[b] (O.D. at 280 mμ)	Specific binding activity (dpm/O.D.)
Untreated plasma	15,500	2.8	5,500
Treated plasma	3,380	2.6	1,300
Control plasma[c]	13,500	2.4	5,600
TeBG fraction	2,380	0.015	159,000

[a]Bound and free steroid separated by gel filtration.
[b]Based on 0.5 ml samples.
[c]Plasma passed through ordinary agarose under otherwise identical conditions.

The protein concentrations were estimated by ultraviolet absorption at 280 mμ and the ratio of bound radioactivity to optical density used as a measure of binding activity. There was a slight decrease in protein content of the treated plasma along with a marked decrease in bound steroid. In terms of ratios, this amounts to a 75 percent loss of TeGB activity. A control experiment where plasma was treated with ordinary agarose under identical conditions showed no significant change in binding of testosterone.

The expected efficiency of the adsorbent was much higher; in fact, a complete separation had been anticipated. Several factors may have prevented this. First, equilibrium conditions probably were not reached because of rapid flow rates. Secondly, it is not known whether all of the steroid on the adsorbent is readily available for binding of the TeBG. In actuality, there may only be a very few active sites on the column.

Elution of the TeBG could not be accomplished either by washing with large volumes of 0.15 M phosphate buffer at pH 7.4 or by lowering the pH to 3.5. Concentrated solutions of guanidine have been used by others (Cuatrecasas and Wilchek, 1968) to release enzymes from insolubilized substrates by reversible denaturation. A 1 M solution of guanidine at pH 2.1 was passed through the adsorbent-TeBG complex and the eluent immediately diluted and neutralized with buffer to pH 7.4. All of the guanidine was removed by gel filtration since it was expected that even traces might interfere with the binding assay. A small amount of binding with testosterone was observed in the treated eluent. The ratio of radioactivity to optical density clearly shows a high degree of purification; however, the yield is quite small.

Improved eluting conditions have not been found as yet. It is interesting to note that others (Vonderhaar and Mueller, 1969) have had the same difficulties using adsorbents with the estrogen-receptor proteins. Perhaps the steroid-binding proteins are unique and will require a different approach for their successful elution.

ANTI-ESTRADIOL ANTIBODY SEPARATION

Estradiol contains the same C and D ring structure as testosterone, so it was thought that this immunosorbent could be used to purify estrogen antibodies. A sample of such an antiserum which had been induced by 17β-succinyl estradiol linked to bovine serum albumin was obtained from Dr. Thorneycroft. This material was derived from a high-titer sheep serum by removal of most of the nonspecific proteins as described earlier in this symposium (Thorneycroft et al., 1970).

When an aliquot of a one-fifth dilution of this antiserum was passed through a column of adsorbent, approximately 80 percent of the protein

TABLE 2

Adsorption of Anti-Estradiol Antibodies by the Immunosorbent

	Protein concentration (O.D. at 280 mμ/unit vol.)	Binding activity[a] (% bound)
Partly purified antiserum[b]	1.83	21.3
Eluted antiserum	0.300	12.4

[a]Measured by a solid-phase assay. Abraham (1969). J. Clin. Endocr., 29:866-870.
[b]Rivanol-treated, anti-BSA precipitated sheep serum, from Thorneycroft et al., 1970.

was held back as measured by the ultraviolet absorption at 280 mμ (Table 2). There was also a correspondingly large decrease in the titer of the eluent using the solid-phase assay system described by Abraham (1969). Washing with relatively large volumes of water or phosphate buffer at pH 6.8 failed to elute any of the antibodies.

It was reasoned that since the antibodies probably have more than one estradiol site per molecule, and since only one site is needed for binding to the immunosorbent, they should exhibit an affinity for estradiol while on the column. When high-specific-activity estradiol in buffer solution was passed through the column, a large proportion of the radioactivity was not eluted (Table 3). A control experiment with the adsorbent unexposed to antibody showed no retention of radioactivity.

TABLE 3

Binding Behavior of the Antibody-Immunosorbent Complex

Substance applied	Amount (dpm)	Eluted radioactivity (dpm)
H^3-estradiol[a]	87,700	24,500
H^3-estradiol (control)[b]	41,600	39,400
H^3-estradiol, then estradiol (10 μg)	95,500	61,900
H^3-estradiol, then testosterone (10 μg)	100,000	4,600

[a]Specific activity 50 C/m$\underline{M}$.
[b]H^3-estradiol was passed through a column of adsorbent with no antibody present.

If the antibody-steroid complex were behaving in a normal manner, then relatively large amounts of unlabeled estradiol should displace the tritiated material. This, in fact, proved to be the case showing that viable protein was on the column. To demonstrate that the antibodies themselves had not been displaced, the eluent from this last experiment was treated with dextran-coated charcoal under conditions known to adsorb only unbound steroid. When this was done all of the radioactivity was removed from solution.

Testosterone is known not to cross-react with this antibody (Thorneycroft et al., 1970) ; therefore, elution with testosterone should not result in displacement of estradiol from the column. Unlabeled testosterone was passed through a column containing the antibody-tritiated estradiol complex. Only a small amount of radioactivity was displaced (Table 3). Whether this represents a measure of cross-reaction is difficult to say because of the excessive amounts being used.

CONCLUSIONS

At this time it is difficult to say how useful this method of purifying proteins will be in the steroid field. It certainly could be applied for the removal of unwanted binding proteins or cross-reacting antibodies from mixtures. This might be important in certain analytic applications.

The observation that the anti-estrogen antibody is an active binding agent, while itself bound to the immunosorbent, could perhaps be the basis for a solid-phase assay. Similar systems have been developed for the routine measurement of luteinizing hormone; however, there the partially purified antibody was chemically bonded to the polysaccharide (Wide and Porath, 1966). Permanent attachment of the anti-estradiol antibody could be achieved by a cross-linking agent, thereby removing the danger of antibody elution. This approach is being investigated to determine if binding activity is unaltered by such treatment. If this turns out to be the case, one could visualize a single column of constant activity being used repetitively for a number of assays.

REFERENCES

Abraham, G. E. 1969. Solid-phase radioimmunoassay of estradiol-17β. J. Clin. Endocr., 29:866–870.

Axen, R., J. Porath, and S. Ernbach. 1967. Chemical coupling of peptides and proteins to polysaccharides by means of cyanogen halides. Nature (London), 214:1302–1304.

Bauminger, S., H. R. Lindner, E. Perel, and R. Arnon. 1969. Antibodies to a phyto-oestrogen: antigenicity of genistein coupled to a synthetic polypeptide. J. Endocr., 44:567–578.

Cuatrecasas, P., and M. Wilchek. 1968. Single-step purification of avidin from egg white by affinity chromatography on biocytin-sepharsoe columns. Biochem. Biophys. Res. Commun., 33:235–239.

———— M. Wilchek, and C. B. Anfinsen. 1968. Selective enzyme purification by affinity chromatography. Proc. Nat. Acad. Sci. USA, 61: 636–643.

Heyns, W., H. van Baelen, and P. de Moor. 1969. Study of the specificity of the steroid-binding-β-globulin in human plasma. J. Endocr., 43:67–71.

Jensen, E. V., E. R. de Sombre, and P. W. Jungblut. 1967. Interaction of estrogens with receptor sites in vivo and in vitro. 2nd Internatl. Congr. Hormonal Steroids, Milan, 1966. Amsterdam, Excerpta Medica Foundation, pp. 492–500.

Landsteiner, K., and J. van der Scheer. 1936. On cross reaction of immune sera to azoproteins. J. Exp. Med., 63:325–339.

Murphy, B. E. P. 1968. Binding of testosterone and estradiol in plasma. Canad. J. Biochem., 46:299–302.

Porath, J., R. Axen, and S. Ernbach. 1967. Chemical coupling of proteins to agarose. Nature (London), 215:1491–1492.

Silman, I. H., and E. Katchalski. 1966. Water insoluble derivatives of enzymes, antigens and antibodies. Ann. Rev. Biochem., 35:873–908.

Thorneycroft, I. H., S. A. Tillson, R. J. Scaramuzzi, G. E. Abraham, and B. V. Caldwell. 1970. Preparation and purification of antibodies to steroids. *In* Péron, F. G., and B. V. Caldwell, eds. Immunologic Methods in Steroid Determination. New York, Appleton-Century-Crofts.

Vermeulen, A., and L. Verdonck. 1968. Studies on the binding of testosterone to human plasma. Steroids, 2:609–635.

Vonderhaar, B., and G. C. Mueller, 1969. Binding of estrogen receptor to estradiol immobilized on insoluble resins. Biochim. Biophys. Acta, 176:626–631.

Wide, L., and J. Porath. 1966. Radioimmunoassay of proteins with the use of Sephadex-coupled antibodies. Biochem. Biophys. Acta, 130: 257–260.

DISCUSSION

W. SLAUNWHITE. We tried much the same experiment with cortisol, using an adduct of cortisol with the copolymer of vinyl chloride and maleic anhydride. We found, as you did, that the transcortin was absorbed out quite well, but we could not get it back in good yield, and therefore gave up this approach. One of the things we did notice (and others have noticed this in other applications) was that if the elution was tried in the presence of an excess of the ligand (steroid) some stability was conferred. I was wondering, when you eluted with guanidine hydrochloride, did you have any ligand present in an attempt to stabilize the protein?

S. BURSTEIN. No, there was no free steroid present. However, this is a possibility that we have to look into.

L. GOODFRIEND.   Is there some way you could test the immunogenicity of your agarose-steroid preparation? It has been our experience, in trying to elute the easily denatured human-reaginic-type antibodies from specific immunosorbents, that 2 M potassium thiocyanate is very effective. You accomplish a clean elution with relatively little denaturation as judged by biologic activity of the eluted antibodies.

S. BURSTEIN.   Is this a specifically anti-steroid antibody?

L. GOODFRIEND.   These are the reaginic, IgE type of antibodies. Thiocyanate elution might work for anti-steroid antibodies, but the nature of the interaction of the steroids with the antibody site might require a qualitatively different type of eluting solvent.

S. BURSTEIN.   In answer to your question whether we tested the agarose-steroid complex for immunogenicity, the physical nature of the substance would make this difficult, since it is essentially a gel and would be difficult to inject.

L. GOODFRIEND.   You can inject the agarose-steroid gel intramuscularly after it has been homogenized.

PART III
The Use of Antibodies to Steroids in Physiologic Studies

10

PHYSIOLOGIC STUDIES
USING ANTIBODIES TO STEROIDS

Burton V. Caldwell, Rex J. Scaramuzzi,
Stephen A. Tillson, Ian H. Thorneycroft
Worcester Foundation for Experimental Biology
Shrewsbury, Massachusetts

INTRODUCTION

Following the comprehensive presentation of Dr. Lieberman et al. in 1959 on the "Chemical, Immunological, and Endocrinological Properties of Steroid-Protein Conjugates," several investigators have described studies utilizing the ability of steroids, when coupled to a carrier protein, to act as haptens and elicit the formation of specific antibodies in properly immunized animals. The previous papers in this symposium have dealt with the chemical and immunologic aspects of steroid-protein conjugates and the reader is referred to these publications for a detailed review of the pertinent literature (Goodfriend and Sehon, 1970; Gross, 1970; Thorneycroft et al., 1970; Pressman and Grossberg, 1970). The primary emphasis of this paper will be on the endocrinologic aspects and the possible use of active and passive immunization procedures in physiologic studies. In particular, evidence will be presented which will more clearly establish the role of estradiol in the control of luteinizing hormone (LH) secretion from the pituitary gland.

Other workers have used passive immunization procedures in attempts to neutralize the effects of endogenous and exogenous steroids in suitable test animals. Neri et al. (1964) reported that antibodies to

This work was supported by NIH training grant 5-T01-AMO 5564-13, the Ford Foundation, and the Agency for International Development.

testosterone could inhibit the biologic effects when testosterone was exogenously administered to castrate rats, as determined by the ratio of seminal vesicle weights to final body weights. The same authors in a similar study showed an inhibition of the effects of exogenous aldosterone after passive immunization with antibodies to aldosterone in adrenalectomized rats, using the ratio of Na to K concentration as the specific bioassay parameter. The neutralization capabilities of antibodies to cortisol were also demonstrated by measuring the effect of this immunization on the number of circulating eosinophils in adrenalectomized rats. For assessing the effects of antibodies to estrone, the same workers used the ratio of uterine weight to final body weight of immature mice to conclude in this case also that the passive immunization procedures were able to neutralize the physiologic effects of exogenously administered estrone. Goodfriend and Sehon (1961) reported previously that antiserum to estrone could neutralize the 6-hour uterotropic activity of exogenous estrone in immature rats, and furthermore showed that the conjugate estrone-17-carbamido-protein was devoid of estrogenic activity on its own. Goodfriend et al. (1961) also reported that by "tagging" the antiserum with fluorescein it was possible to localize, in the ovary of the mature rat, cellular components which cross-reacted with the fluorescein-labeled antiserum to estrone-2-carbamido-HSA. Recently Ferin et al. (1968, 1969) have extended the previous work showing that the passive immunization with antiserum to estradiol inhibited the biologic effects of estradiol administered to immature and mature ovariectomized rats and mice. They also reported that the antiserum prevented the uterine weight increases, endometrial stimulation, and vaginal cornification due to endogenous estrogens following treatment with human chorionic gonadotropin (HCG). Pretreatment of intact animals with the antisera inhibited the uptake of tritiated estradiol by the uteri, pituitaries, and ovaries. Diethylstilbestrol (DES), a synthetic estrogen, was shown by them to retain its estrogenic activity in the passively immunized animals. In immature rats the administration of antiserum to estradiol up to 15 hours prior to the expected time of LH release blocked ovulation in PMS-treated (Pregnant Mares' Serum) immature rats. Since the injection of HCG restored ovulation in the immunized animals, it was reasoned that the responsiveness of the ovaries to the gonadotropin was unaffected by the antiserum, and these authors concluded that the antibodies to estradiol acted by suppressing LH release. They were also able to replace the "blocked" endogenous estrogen with exogenous DES, although they recorded only a 30 to 40 percent incidence of ovulation following the injection of different doses of DES. The details of these and further studies will be presented by Ferin et al. (1970) in the following paper, therefore no additional analysis of their work will be considered here.

EFFECTS OF ACTIVE AND PASSIVE IMMUNIZATION AGAINST ESTRADIOL IN THE CYCLING HAMSTER

All of the above studies used passive immunization procedures to attempt the neutralization of the physiologic effects of exogenous and, in some cases, endogenous steroids. Our approach to these studies was to actively immunize various animals against estradiol-17β (estradiol) for use in the physiologic studies, reasoning that we should achieve the highest titer of antibodies in actively immunized animals. The principal aim was to examine the factors influencing ovarian periodicity as related to the circulating level of estradiol. We selected, therefore, a simplified test system which would allow us to measure the alteration of ovarian periodicity as influenced by the immunization procedures.

The estrous cycle of the golden hamster has a very reliable duration of 4 days (Deanesly, 1938) and is characterized by the lack of a fully functional corpus luteum unless sterile or fertile mating has occurred on the day of overt estrous behavior. We selected as our specific parameter the appearance of the characteristic lordosis response which occurs on only one day (hereafter called day 4) of the estrous cycle. The female hamster is a very pugnacious animal and on the other 3 days of the cycle she is anything but receptive to a male of the species. The animals were caged individually in a reversed lighting room for the convenience of the investigators, and every morning a male was placed in each female's cage while observations were made on the behavioral response of both animals. Each of the experimental animals was allowed at least three cycles of normal duration prior to being placed into one of three groups at random. Of the 90 control cycles observed, 100 percent were of the normal 4-day duration, attesting to the extreme reliability of this method for measuring the estrous interval (Table 1).

TABLE 1

The Effects of Immunization Against Estradiol in the Cycling Hamster

Group	No. of cycles observed		Length of cycles (days)						% Normal cycles	
	Before	After	Before			After			Before	After
			<4	4	>4	<4	4	>4		
Control[a]	18	60	0	18	0	0	58	2	100	97
Active[b]	36	142	0	36	0	56	70	16	100	49[d]
Passive[c]	36	62	0	36	0	4	41	17	100	65[d]

[a]Freund's complete adjuvant in saline.
[b]BSA-estradiol-17β.
[c]Sheep antisera to estradiol-17β.
[d]Treatments significantly different from controls (P< .005).

The animals in the control group were immunized with Freund's complete adjuvant emulsified in a 1:1 mixture with sterile saline (1 ml/animal) injected into five subcutaneous sites once a week for 4 weeks and monthly thereafter with the same dosage. Of 60 cycles observed following this immunization, only two were elongated (both 5 days) which can be contrasted with the results from the animals actively immunized against estradiol. The only difference in the procedures for the first two groups was the addition of 1 mg of the estradiol 17β-bovine serum albumin conjugate (E-2-BSA) to the emulsion that was injected. Of the 142 cycles measured after this immunization, only 56 were of normal length with the predominant alteration being to shortened cycles. In fact, it was not uncommon for individual animals to show several 2-day estrous cycles in a row followed often by a significantly elongated cycle. This is an extremely unlikely occurrence under natural conditions. The animals which were immunized passively received partially purified antibodies prepared in the following manner. Antisera produced in sheep to E-2-BSA was adsorbed free of the antibodies directed against the natural hapten groups present on the BSA molecule and treated with Rivanol in a manner described by Thorneycroft et al. (1970). This removed most of the serum proteins that were not gamma globulins. After freeze drying, 3 mg of this antibody-containing fraction were administered in 1 ml saline by intraperitoneal injection of every day for 7 days and weekly thereafter. Table 1 shows clearly that, once again, ovarian periodicity was altered although not to the same extent as found following active immunization. In this case, however, the predominant alteration in cycle length was to a longer duration.

Both of the experimental groups differed significantly from the controls (Students' t test) (Table 1). However, we were unable to specifically delineate the possible mechanism by which the immunizations had caused such severe alteration of the cycle. We lacked the methodology to measure a more precise parameter in the hamster, and therefore shifted our studies to measurement of LH in the ewe, since Scaramuzzi et al., (1970) had finished the developmental stages of a radioimmunoassay for ovine LH.

THE EFFECTS OF ACTIVE IMMUNIZATION AGAINST ESTRADIOL 17-β IN THE OVARIECTOMIZED EWE

All of the details for the radioimmunoassay method of ovine LH (double-antibody separation of free from bound) used for these studies will be reported in a future publication (Scaramuzzi et al., 1970). However, for the purpose of indicating the reliability of the method, Table 2 shows the values recorded for LH on seven different occasions using the same high LH level plasma pool. This was necessary since the

TABLE 2

Reproducibility of LH Levels from a Plasma Pool

Assay no.	Date	Number	Concentration of LH (ng NIH-S11/ml)
1	Aug. 25	20	10.11
2	Aug. 26	3	12.00
3	Aug. 28	3	12.25
4	Sept. 24	3	9.25
5	Oct. 10	3	11.25
6	Oct. 14	3	9.50
7	Oct. 15	3	12.00

Mean $\pm$ SE: 10.91 $\pm$ 0.48 (7 assays, 38 determinations).
Coefficient of variation 11.40%.

determinations of LH from our experimental animals were performed over a period of several months and some measure of the consistency of the method had to be attempted so that comparisons could be made between the levels recorded from the individual assays. Throughout the duration of the experiments, a mean value of 10.91 $\pm$ 0.48 ng/ml ($\pm$ SE) of LH in the plasma pool was estimated with a coefficient of variation of 11.40 percent, which is well within the accepted range for precision of a radioimmunoassay.

In order to simplify our test system, we used ovariectomized ewes and followed a protocol established by Robinson (1959) to simulate the natural sequence of steroids usually present during a normal estrous cycle of intact ewes. Figure 1 gives the details for the procedure wherein 20 mg

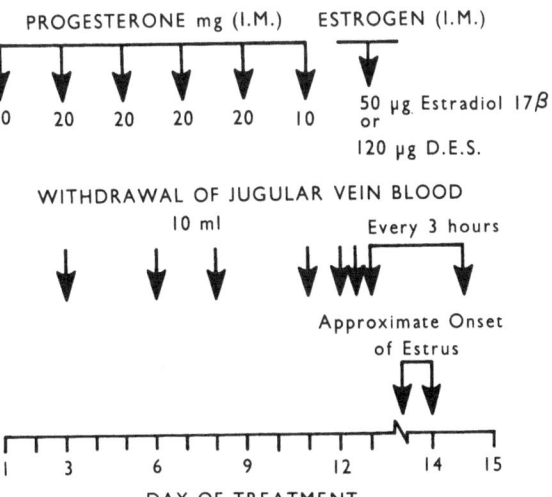

Fig. 1. Experimental protocol for inducing behavioral estrus in ovariectomized ewes. All steroids administered in oil by intramuscular injection. DES is diethylstilbestrol.

of progesterone in oil was administered every other day beginning on day 1 of the induced estrous cycle for a period of 10 days. On day 11, 10 mg of progesterone was administered (all steroids given by intramuscular injection; IM) followed 2 days later by the injection of an estrogen in quantities as shown. This sequence is approximately in keeping with the normal secretory pattern of the main steroids produced by the sheep ovary as reported in several papers (Short et al., 1963; Plotka and Erb, 1967; Moore et al., 1969). Essentially this procedure was used recently by Radford et al. (1969) to demonstrate that the peak level of LH occurred approximately 24 hours after the injection of estradiol benzoate. The onset and duration of estrus was also measured and found to be normal following this injection schedule. Other investigations have also reported on LH levels in the ewe, and generally agree that the peak of LH follows the onset of estrus by 4 to 24 hours (Niswender et al., 1968; Dierschke and Clegg, 1968; Goding et al., 1969; Geschwind and Dewey, 1968; Wheatley and Radford, 1969). All of the above studies added to the growing weight of indirect evidence that the increase of estradiol which occurs prior to the rise of LH may be responsible for causing the release of this presumably "ovulatory" hormone, and the present experiments were designed specifically to examine this relationship. As depicted in Figure 1, 10 ml of jugular vein blood was collected periodically during the progesterone treatment and every 3 hours following the estrogen injection. This blood was heparinized, centrifuged, and stored at −4°C until ready for assay.

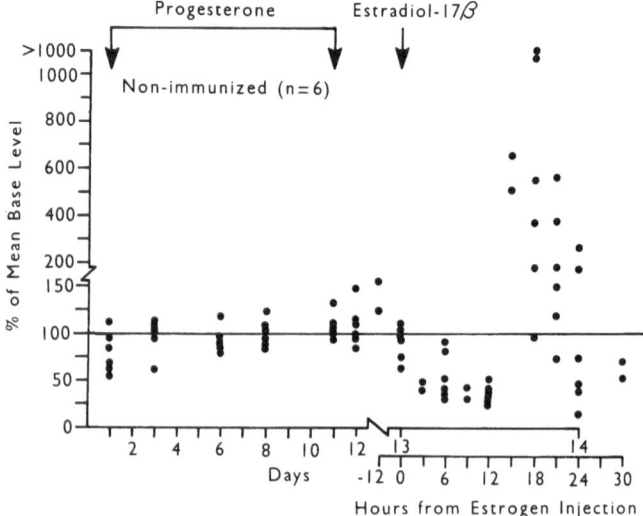

Fig. 2. LH levels in nonimmunized ovariectomized ewes. Each dot represents the percent of the mean base level which was calculated as the mean of LH measured for each animal throughout the progesterone-treatment period.

Figure 2 shows the LH levels of control animals treated with 50 µg estradiol after the progesterone injections. In order to present the results in a uniform fashion, the actual mass of LH found in each blood collection was transformed to percent of mean base level to show the general trends of LH levels. The mean base level was calculated as the mean of LH values measured during the progesterone-treatment period. It is obvious from these results that LH levels tend to fall 6 to 12 hours after estradiol administration and rapidly increase to peak levels approximately 18 hours post-injection. This is in sharp contrast to the pattern seen in Figure 3, following the same procedure but using ewes previously immunized against estradiol by the following procedure. In a 5-ml emulsion of Freund's complete adjuvant and saline, (v:v) 3 mg of the E-2-BSA complex was dissolved and injected into five subcutaneous sites once a week for 6 weeks and monthly thereafter for at least 4 months (Thorneycroft et al., 1970). The result of this immunization procedure was to completely neutralize the stimulation of LH secretion from the pituitary, since there was no significant variation from the mean base level throughout the treatment period. The tendency for low levels of LH immediately following the estrogen injection and the peak of LH shortly thereafter, as shown in the control animals, was absent. Proceeding on the assumption that it was the high titer of antibodies to estradiol which "bound" the estradiol in the general circulation resulting in the neutralization of the physiologic effects normally found following estradiol injection, the titer and affinity of the antisera collected from the immunized animals were determined using the solid-phase system

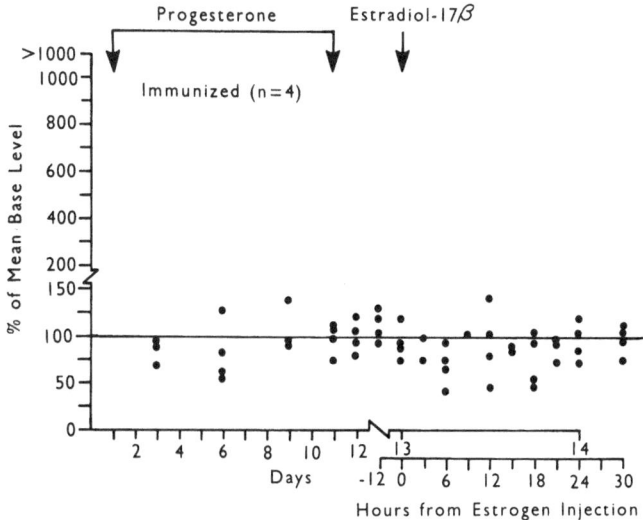

Fig. 3. LH levels in ovariectomized ewes immunized against estradiol-17β. (See Figs. 1 and 2 for further details.)

described by Abraham (1969a) and Tillson et al. (1970). The results of this in vitro analysis showed the titer to be very high (1:10,000 dilution gave a 50 percent binding of tritiated estradiol) and the affinity to be so high as to make extraction of labeled estradiol from the antisera nearly impossible using standard solvent extraction techniques. The in vitro studies provided an opportunity to test the ability of the antisera to estradiol to bind DES, since, as mentioned previously, other investigators had used this synthetic estrogen to overcome the block of estradiol noted after passive immunization (Ferin et al., 1969). Using the procedure described by Tillson et al. (1970) it was found that DES was bound less than 0.1 percent when compared to estradiol binding by the same antisera. Robinson (1961) had used DES in progesterone-primed spayed ewes and demonstrated that this estrogenlike compound was very effective in inducing behavioral estrus. We reasoned that the behavioral effect most likely indicated that LH release had also been stimulated by the administration of DES.

When 120 μg of DES was administered instead of estradiol, the pattern of LH levels (Fig. 4) was nearly identical with that of the control animals shown in Figure 2. Both the depression and increase of LH were present following DES administration. The same procedure was then followed using the immunized animals, and for the first time a decrease in LH was recorded followed by a peak level about 12 to 18 hours after the DES injection (Fig. 5), adding direct evidence that the increase in estrogen is responsible for "triggering" the release of LH in sheep. One

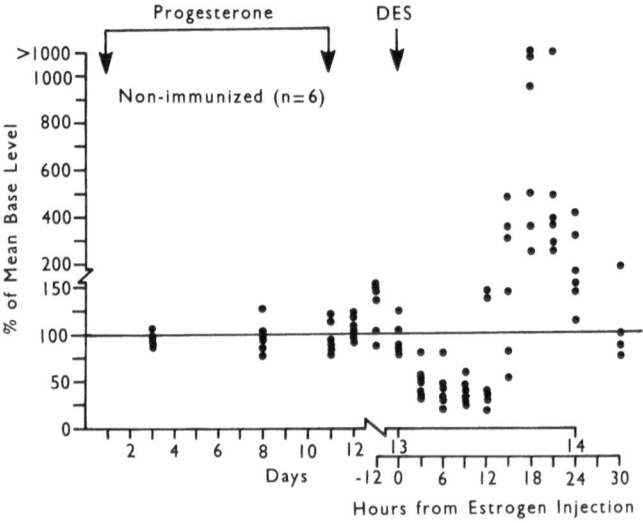

Fig. 4. LH levels in nonimmunized, ovariectomized ewes. (See Figs. 1 and 2 for further details.)

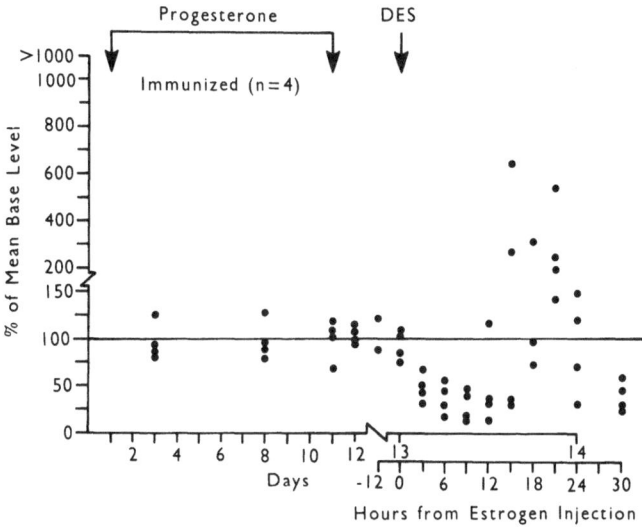

Fig. 5. LH levels in ovariectomized ewes immunized against estradiol-17β. (See Figs. 1 and 2 for further details.)

final control experiment showed that the withdrawal of progesterone, thought by some to be involved in the release of LH, did not by itself have any significant effect on the pattern of LH secretion (Fig. 6).

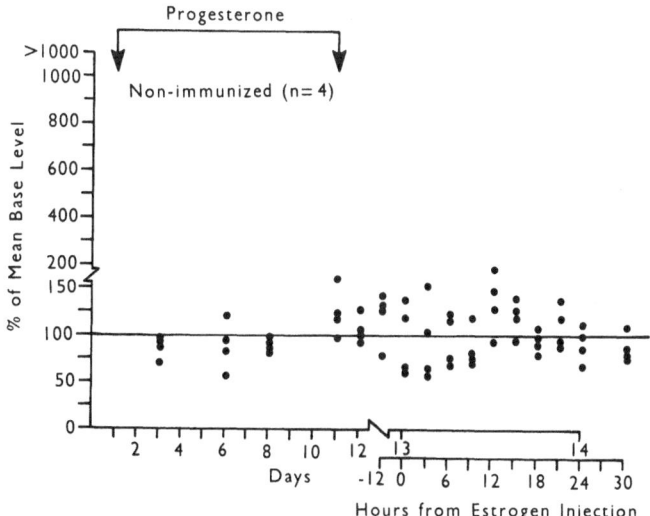

Fig. 6. LH levels in nonimmunized, ovariectomized ewes following progesterone injection. (See text and Figs. 1 and 2 for further details.)

Radford et al. (1969) had previously suggested that the withdrawal of progesterone before the injection of estradiol may be responsible for a slight rise in LH. The fall in progesterone levels coupled with the increase in the estrogen secretion may be the stimulation for the estrus LH peak. The results of the present experiment do not confirm the above concept; however, the interrelationship of progesterone and estradiol in intact animals may be a significant factor in regulating LH secretion.

In an effort to present a succinct summary of the data, Figure 7 shows the mean levels of LH measured throughout the treatment period in control and immunized animals with estradiol injected on day 13. The clear contrast in pattern is self-evident. When compared to the results shown in Figure 8, the most reasonable conclusion is that the estrogen DES was not bound totally by the antibodies to estradiol, and stimulated the secretion or release of LH from the pituitary. Of particular importance also is the significant drop in LH shown following DES administration to the immunized animals, once again duplicating the pattern seen in the control animals.

In sheep, the incidence of behavioral estrus in ovariectomized ewes should be virtually 100 percent after the experimental protocol followed in the present study and indeed, all of the control animals showed normal behavioral responses when either estradiol or DES was injected. However, only two of the immunized animals showed any signs of estrus following estradiol injection, and the onset and duration were very

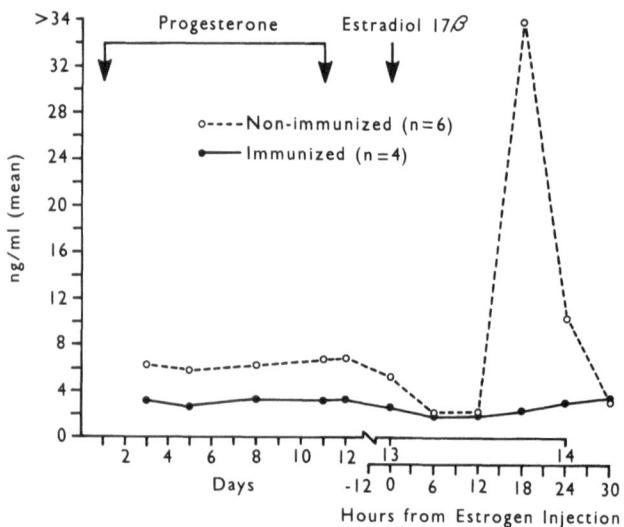

Fig. 7. Mean LH levels in control and immunized ovariectomized ewes following injection of progesterone and estradiol-17β. (See Fig. 1.)

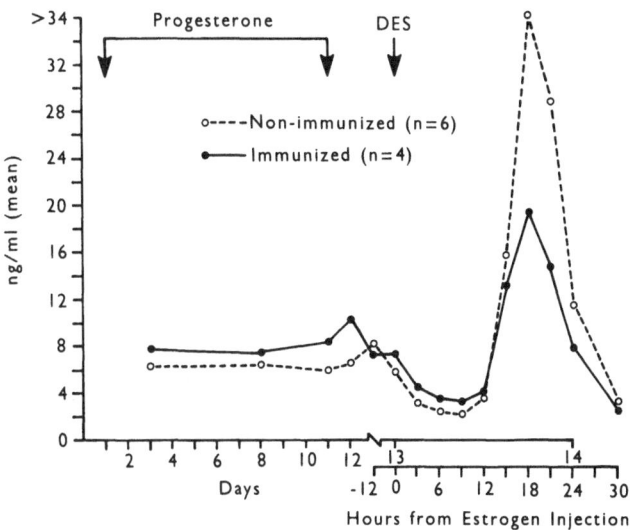

Fig. 8. Mean LH levels in control and immunized ovariectomized ewes following injection of progesterone and diethylstilbestrol (See Fig. 1.)

abnormal. This is in contrast to the 100 percent incidence of behavioral response shown by the same immunized animals after administration of DES. None of the animals receiving progesterone only showed any signs characteristic of estrus. Estrous behavior was detected by individual observation of each experimental animal in the presence of a vasectomized ram fitted with a harness containing a marking crayon for recording the mounting of the ewe.

DISCUSSION

The results of the above investigation when added to the rather large body of data reported by others provide the basis for our conclusion that the stimulation of LH release in the ewe prior to ovulation is due to the great increase in estradiol-17β which usually occurs about 24 hours prior to the peak of LH. The many consistencies between the pattern of steroid secretion and gonadotropin levels in the human and sheep suggest the possible extrapolation of the above conclusion to the human. It has been shown by Baird and Guevara (1969) that the midcycle peak concentration of LH in plasma corresponded with the maximum concentration of estradiol in seven women subjects. However, the sampling procedure would not have permitted a more close approximation of the exact relationship between the two hormones. Recently, the exact sequence of estradiol and LH has been suggested by several authors (Abraham, 1969b; Korenman et al., 1969; Goebelsmann et al., 1969; and Corker et al., 1969). All have reported that the peak of LH followed the highest level of estradiol by about a day. Swerdloff and Odell (1968) have discussed in detail the possible feedback mechanisms which may be operating to regulate the cyclic variation in LH levels in women and have suggested that either a rise in a progestogen or estrogen might account for the LH surge. Concerning the progestogen possibility, it is pertinent to note the concomitant rise of LH and 17-hydroxyprogesterone in women reported by Strott et al. (1969). However, these authors do not suggest that LH release is necessarily a function of the increased secretion of 17-hydroxyprogesterone.

The relationship between estradiol and FSH is another complex subject and will not be treated here in detail. However, since both LH and FSH appear to rise together in the human, and since FSH may perhaps rise prior to LH in sheep (Robertson, 1966), the definitive relationship between these gonadotropins and estradiol remains to be elucidated. Our present studies are designed to examine this point and our primary efforts are directed toward the development of a radioimmunoassay for ovine FSH. Duplicate blood samples were taken throughout the entire range of experiments reported on the ovariectomized sheep used in this paper, and an analysis of the effects of immunization against estradiol on FSH levels would complement our reported observations on LH levels following this procedure.

Ferin et al. (1970) will discuss other possible applications of immunologic techniques in physiologic studies in the following paper, obviating the presentation of similar speculation here. However, it should be noted that the general principle of immunologic approaches need not be confined to the study of reproductive processes and significant advances might be expected from the application of these techniques to other areas of current interest. The physiologic neutralization of various steroids by passive and active immunization might be an important tool in the possible control of some steroid-susceptible cancers, cancers which tend to regress following gonadectomy or hypophysectomy. Of possible importance also is the general application of the radioimmunoassay described by several workers in this symposium to other nonsteroidal, small-molecular-weight substances which could also act as haptens. In particular, methods are critically needed for estimating the circulating levels of drugs such as the cannabinols and morphine. Both these substances have the chemical characteristics which would permit their conjugation to protein carriers for immunization procedures.

It would appear that a potentially valuable tool has become available to the investigator in bio-medical sciences, the real value of which depends upon the ultimate imagination of the individual and his application of the techniques in developing new methodology in the examination of physiologic processes.

Acknowledgments

The authors gratefully acknowledge the assistance of Miss Miriam Kangas, Mr. Lawrence Underwood, and Dr. John McCracken.

REFERENCES

Abraham, G. E. 1969a. Solid-phase radioimmunoassay of estradiol 17-beta. J. Clin. Endocr., 29:866–870.

———— 1969b. Plasma immunoreactive estrogens and L.H. during the menstrual cycle. (Abstract). Proc. of Fifty-first Meet. Endocr. Soc., p. 115.

Baird, D. T., and A. Guevara. 1969. Concentration of unconjugated estrone and estradiol in peripheral plasma in nonpregnant women throughout the menstrual cycle, castrate and postmenopausal women and in men. J. Clin. Endocr., 29:149–156.

Brown, J. M., K. J. Catt, I. A. Cumming, J. R. Goding, C. C. Kaltenbach, and B. J. Mole. 1969. The release of luteinizing hormone in the ewe following oestradiol administration. Proc. Physiol. Soc., 201:98–100.

Corker, C. S., F. Naftolin, and D. Exley. 1969. Interrelationship between plasma luteinizing hormone and oestradiol in the human menstrual cycle. Nature (London), 222:1063.

Deansly, R. 1938. The reproductive cycle of the golden hamster (Cricetus Auratus). Proc. Zool. Soc. London (Series A), 108:31–37.

Dierschke, D. J., and M. T. Clegg. 1968. Studies on the relationship of serum and pituitary gonadotropin levels to ovulation in the ewe. J. Reprod. Fertil., 15:321–324.

Ferin, M., P. E. Zimmering, and R. L. Vande Wiele. 1969. Effects of antibodies to estradiol-17β on PMS-induced ovulation in immature rats. Endocrinology, 84:893–900.

———— J. Raziano, A. Tempone, and R. L. Vande Wiele. 1970. The use of antibodies as a tool in the study of reproductive physiology. *In* Péron, F. G., and B. V. Caldwell, eds. Immunologic Methods in Steroid Determination. New York, Appleton-Century-Crofts.

———— P. E. Zimmering, S. Lieberman, and R. L. Vande Wiele. 1968. Inactivation of the biological effects of exogenous and endogenous estrogens by antibodies to 17β-estradiol. Endocrinology, 83:565–571.

Geschwind, I. I., and R. Dewey. 1968. Dynamics of luteinizing hormone secretion in the cycling ewe: a radioimmunoassay study. P.S.E.B.M., 129:451–455.

Goding, J. R., K. J. Catt, J. M. Brown, C. C. Kaltenbach, I. A. Cumming, and B. J. Mole. 1969. Radioimmunoassay for ovine luteinizing hormone during estrus and following estrogen administration in the sheep. Endocrinology, 85:133–142.

Goebelsmann, U., A. R. Midgley, and R. R. Jaffe. 1969. Regulation of human gonadotropins. VII. Daily individual urinary estrogens, pregnanediol and serum luteinizing and follicle stimulating hormones during the menstrual cycle. J. Clin. Endocr., 29:1222–1230.

Goodfriend, L., and A. H. Sehon. 1970. Early approaches to production, analysis and use of steroid-specific antisera. In Péron, F. G., and B. V. Caldwell, eds. Immunologic Methods in Steroid Determination. New York, Appleton-Century-Crofts.

———— and A. H. Sehon. 1961. Antibodies to estrone protein conjugates. II. Endocrinological studies. Canad. J. Biochem. Physiol., 39:962–965.

———— A. M. Leznoff, and A. H. Sehon. 1961. Antibodies to estrone-protein conjugates. III. Tissue localization of estrogens. Canad. J. Biochem. Physiol., 39:967–971.

Gross, S. 1970. Specification of steroid antibodies. In Péron, F. G., and B. V. Caldwell, eds. Immunologic Methods in Steroid Determination. New York, Appleton-Century-Crofts.

Korenman, S., L. Perrin, and B. Rao. 1969. Menstrual variation of the plasma estradiol: Demonstration of elevation prior to the ovulatory LH peak. (Abstract). Proc. Fifty-first Meet. Endocr. Soc., p. 115.

Lieberman, S., F. Erlanger, S. M. Beiser, and F. J. Agate, Jr. 1959. Steroid-protein conjugates: their chemical, immuno-chemical, and endocrinological properties. Recent Progr. Hormone Res., 15:165–200.

Moore, N. W., S. Barrett, J. B. Brown, I. Schindler, A. A. Smith and B. Smyth. 1969. Oestrogen and progesterone content of ovarian vein blood of the ewe during the oestrous cycle. J. Endocr., 44:55–62.

Neri, R. O., S. Tolksdorf, S. M. Beiser, B. F. Erlanger, F. J. Agate, Jr., and S. Lieberman. 1964. Further studies on the biological effects of passive immunization to steroid-protein conjugates. Endocrinology, 74:593–598.

Niswender, G. D., J. F. Roche, D. L. Foster, and A. R. Midgley, Jr. 1968. Radioimmunoassay of serum levels of luteinizing hormone during the cycle and early pregnancy in ewes. P.S.E.B.M., 129:901–904.

Plotka, E. D., and R. E. Erb. 1967. Levels of progesterone in peripheral blood plasma during the estrous cycle of the ewe. J. Anim. Sci., 26:1363–1365.

Pressman, D., and A. Grossberg. 1970. Structural basis of antibody specificity. In Péron, F. G., and B. V. Caldwell, eds. Immunologic Methods in Steroid Determination. New York, Appleton-Century-Crofts.

Radford, H. M., I. S. Wheatley, and A. L. C. Wallace. 1969. The effects of oestradiol benzoate and progesterone on secretion of luteinizing hormone in the ovariectomized ewe. J. Endocr., 44:135–136.

Robertson, H. A. 1966. Gonadotrophin secretion in relation to oestrus and to ovulation. In Lamming, G. E., and E. C. Amoroso, eds. Reproduction in the Female Mammal. 195–211, New York, Plenum Press.

Robinson, T. J. 1959. The estrous cycle of the ewe and doe. In Cole, H. H., and P. T. Cupps, eds. Reproduction in Domestic Animals. New York, Academic Press, Inc.

—————— and T. F. Reardon. 1961. The activity of a number of oestrogens as tested in the spayed ewe. J. Endocr., 23:97–107.

Scaramuzzi, R. J., B. V. Caldwell, and R. M. Moor. 1970. Radioimmunoassay of LH and estradiol during the estrous cycle of the ewe. Biology of Reproduction, 3:110–119.

Short, R. V. 1964. Ovarian steroid synthesis and secretion in vivo. Recent Progr. Hormone Res., 20:303–339.

—————— M. F. McDonald, and L. E. A. Rowson. 1963. Steroids in the ovarian venous blood of ewes before and after gonadotropic stimulation. J. Endocr., 26:155–169.

Strott, C. A., T. Yoshimi, G. T. Ross, and M. B. Lipsett. 1969. Ovarian physiology: relationship between plasma LH and steroidogenesis by the follicles and corpus luteum; effect of HCG. J. Clin. Endocr., 29:1157–1167.

Swerdloff, R. S., and W. D. Odell. 1968. Gonadotropins: present concepts in the human. Calif. Med., 109:467–485.

Thorneycroft, I. H., S. A. Tillson, G. E. Abraham, R. S. Scaramuzzi, and B. V. Caldwell. 1970. Preparation and purification of antibodies to steroids. *In* Péron, F. G., and B. V. Caldwell, eds. Immunologic Methods in Steroid Determination. New York, Appleton-Century-Crofts.

Tillson, S. A., I. H. Thorneycroft, G. Abraham, and B. V. Caldwell. 1970. Solid-phase radioimmunoassay of steroids. *In* Péron, F. G., and B. V. Caldwell, eds. Immunologic Methods in Steroid Determination. New York, Appleton-Century-Crofts.

Wheatley, I. S., and H. M. Radford. 1969. Luteinizing hormone secretion during the estrous cycle of the ewe as determined by radioimmunoassay. J. Reprod. Fertil., 19:211–214.

11

THE USE OF ANTIBODIES AS A TOOL IN STUDIES IN REPRODUCTIVE PHYSIOLOGY

Michel Ferin,* Joseph Raziano,† Antonio Tempone,‡ Raymond L. Vande Wiele§

Department of Obstetrics and Gynecology,
Columbia University College of Physicians and Surgeons
New York, New York

INTRODUCTION

In an earlier presentation to this symposium (Mikhail et al., 1970) we have reported the development of a radioimmunoassay method for plasma 17β-estradiol and estrone, a method which involves the use of antibodies to 17β-estradiol produced by the hapten technique. The purpose of this presentation is to describe a series of physiologic studies in which such antibodies to steroids were used as experimental tools to evaluate the role of 17β-estradiol, progesterone and testosterone in various reproductive processes.

The steroid-protein conjugates employed for the production of the antibodies used in the experiments to be described were the following: 17β-estradiol-succinyl-BSA progesterone-20-o-carboxymethyl-oxime-BSA and testosterone-3-o-carboxymethyl-oxime-BSA. For immunization pur-

These studies were supported in part by U.S.P.H.S. grant NO. HD 02996.
* International Institute for the Study of Human Reproduction.
† U.S.P.H.S. Trainee.
‡ Present address: University of Buenos Aires School of Medicine, Argentina.
§ Career Investigator, Health Research Council in the City of New York.

poses the antigens were mixed with an equal volume of Freund's complete adjuvant and injected into adult ewes. The antisera were absorbed with BSA to remove antibodies to this carrier protein, and the concentration of steroid-specific antibodies was quantitated by precipitin curves and expressed as mg/ml (Zimmering et al., 1965). In a few instances, a γ-globulin fraction was prepared and used in the experiments, but in most cases unfractionated antisera were used. In all experiments antibodies were administered intraperitoneally.

NEUTRALIZATION OF EXOGENOUS ESTROGENS

A series of experiments were performed to determine whether antibodies to 17β-estradiol (anti-E_2) would inhibit the biologic effects of exogenous 17β-estradiol (Ferin et al., 1968). Similar studies dealing with antisera produced by immunization with estrone conjugates have been reported (Goodfriend and Sehon, 1961; Neri et al., 1964). Figure 1 illustrates a study of the inhibition by anti-E_2 of the uterotrophic effect of 17β-estradiol. Immature mice were used and the height of each bar indicates uterine weight. Estradiol (0.2 μg) increased the weight of the uterus from a control value of 10 mg to approximately 50 mg. When increasing doses of antibody were injected, there was a progressive decrease in uterine weight. Maximum inhibition was obtained with an amount of antiserum equivalent to 1 mg of antibody, but even at the plateau values the uterine weights were still higher than those of the uninjected controls. These results were not unexpected. It is likely that

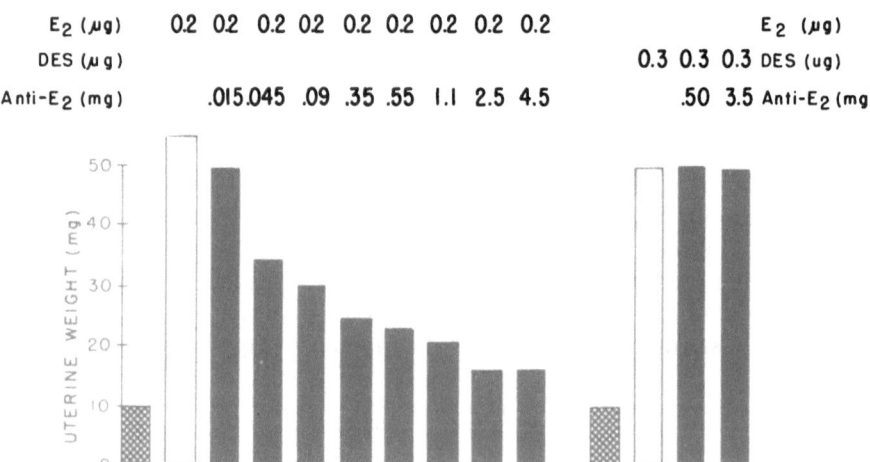

Fig. 1. Effect of administration of anti-E_2 on the uterotrophic activity of 17β-estradiol and diethylstilbestrol (DES).

in view of the nature of the binding of 17β-estradiol to its antibody, a small fraction of the steroid remains free in the circulation even in the presence of excess antibody, making complete inhibition of the estrogen effect impossible. In view of the differences in structure between diethylstilbestrol (DES) and 17β-estradiol, it could be expected that the uterotrophic effect of diethylstilbestrol would not be inhibited by anti-E_2. The results of some experiments, also illustrated in Figure 1, indicate that this hypothesis was indeed correct. A dose of 0.3 µg of DES produced an increase in the uterine weight similar to that of 0.2 µg of 17β-estradiol. Amounts of anti-E_2 which gave maximum suppression of the 17β-estradiol activity did not produce any change in the uterotrophic effect of diethylstilbestrol. In these and subsequently described experiments, there was no evidence that the antisera were in any way toxic, and body weights of the treated and control animals were always identical.

Similar experiments were carried out in adult ovariectomized rats (Ferin et al., 1968). In this species also, the increase in uterine weight

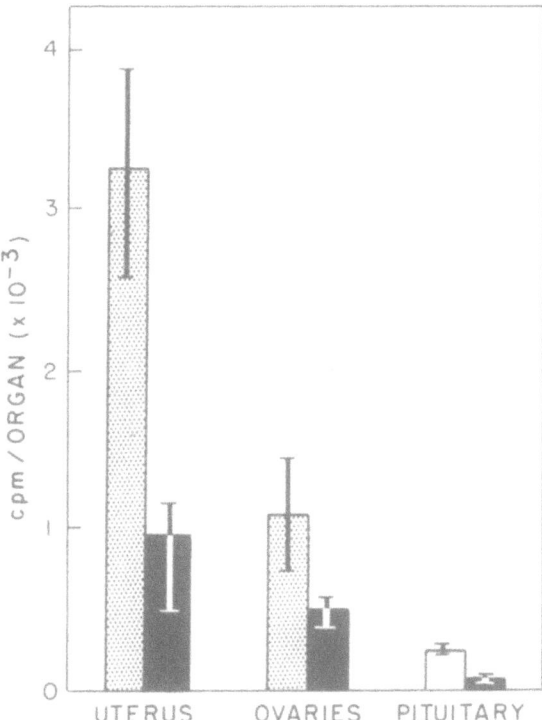

Fig. 2. Total radioactivity (CPM/organ) after injection of 2.3 µc of 17β-estradiol, 6,7-³H into controls and rats pretreated with anti-serum to estradiol (mean ± range). Solid areas are for animals pretreated with anti-E_2. Others are controls. The bars represent average values. The lines show the range within each group.

resulting from the administration of 17β-estradiol was inhibited, as was the proliferation of the endometrium and the vaginal epithelium, with none or very few cornified cells appearing in the vaginal smears of animals injected with anti-E₂.

In 10 immature rats, the uptake of ^{3}H-17β-estradiol by the uterus, ovaries, and pituitary was studied in the presence of antibodies to 17β-estradiol. The amount of ^{3}H-17β-estradiol taken up by these tissues is markedly reduced after treatment with anti-E₂ (Fig. 2). Similar results have been reported after treatment with other estrogen antagonists such as MER 25 and clomiphene citrate (Roy et al., 1964; Jensen, et al., 1964), but the mechanism of action is likely to be different. Antiestrogens such as clomiphene citrate appear to compete with the estrogens for the receptor sites in the uterus, while the anti-E₂ binds the estrogen in the circulation so that less hormone reaches the receptor sites.

The immunologic specificity of the hapten-antibody reaction under in vitro conditions has been the subject of several reports to this symposium. We have carried out a number of experiments to study the specificity of the steroid-antibody reaction under in vivo conditions. Some of these experiments are illustrated in Figures 3 and 4. The experimental conditions were the same as those shown in Figure 1. It is evident that neither antibodies to testosterone (anti-T) or to progesterone (anti-P) had any effect upon the uterotrophic activity of 17β-estradiol. Vice versa, anti-E₂ did not inhibit the increase in weight of the seminal vesicles in testosterone-treated rats.

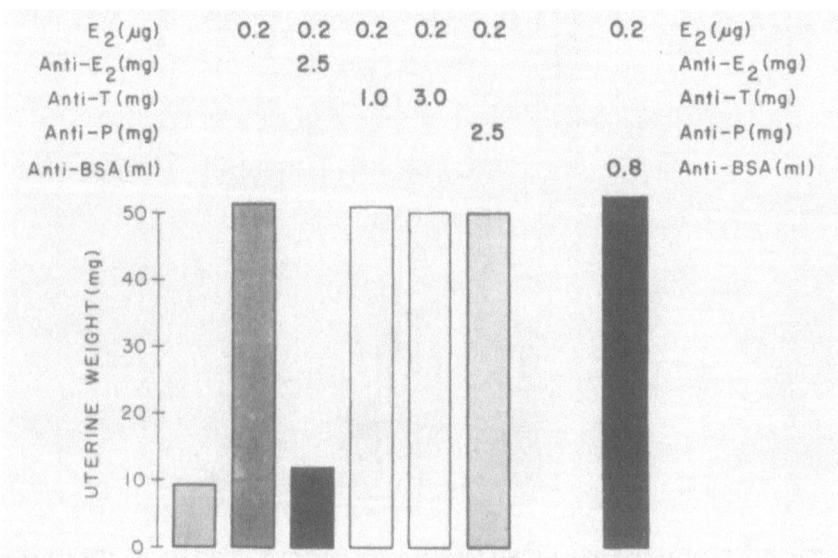

Fig. 3. Effect of antibodies to estradiol, testosterone, progesterone, and BSA on the uterotrophic effect of estradiol.

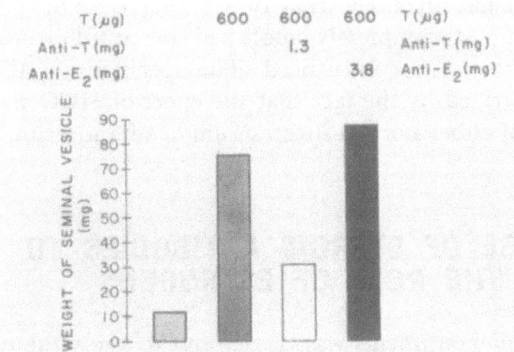

Fig. 4. Effect of testosterone propionate and anti-E₂ on the weight of seminal vesicles in immature rats.

INACTIVATION OF ENDOGENOUS ESTROGENS

Antibodies to 17β-estradiol not only neutralize the biologic activity of exogenous, but also of endogenous estrogens. When 0.5 IU of HCG were administered to immature mice, the ovarian weight doubled and

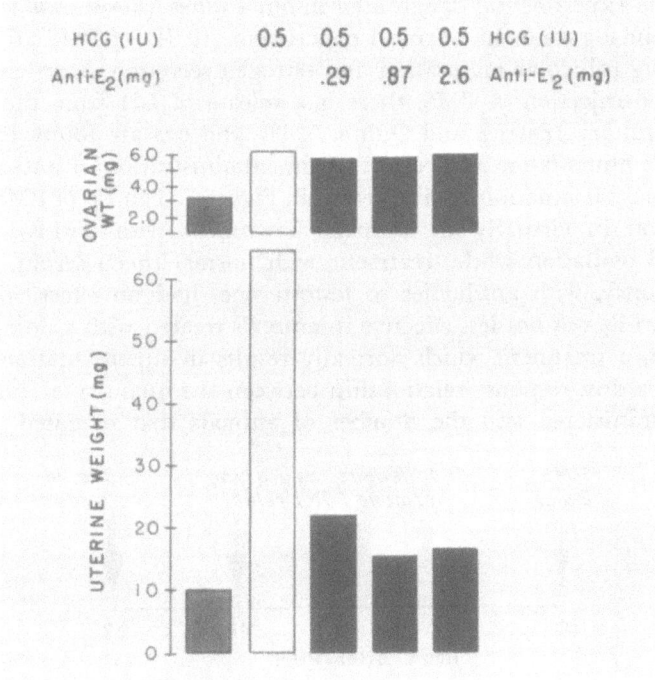

Fig. 5. Effect of HCG and anti-E₂ on the ovarian and uterine weights in immature mice.

the uterine weight increased from 10 to 50 mg (Fig. 5). The effect on the uterus was almost completely abolished by anti-E_2, but, interestingly, ovarian weight was not influenced. The specificity of this reaction was again demonstrated by the fact that the effect of HCG was not inhibited by injection of either normal sheep serum or of antiserum to testosterone.

THE USE OF STEROID ANTIBODIES TO STUDY THE ROLE OF ESTROGENS

A series of experiments was carried out to study the role of estrogens and progesterone as triggers to the preovulatory LH release. Two experimental models were used. In the first set of experiments, the effect of the administration of anti-E_2 on the endogenous LH release of the PMS-treated immature rat was studied. In the second set of experiments, anti-E_2 and anti-P were administered to 4-day cyclic rats and the results of such treatment upon LH release and ovulation were evaluated.

The PMS-treated Rat

The experimental design used in our studies (Ferin et al., 1969a) is shown in Figure 6. In a typical experiment, 10 IU of PMS are injected, initiating follicular maturation and estrogen secretion. Forty-eight hours after the injection of PMS, there is a release of LH from the animal's own pituitary (Zarrow and Quinn, 1963) and ova are found in the oviducts 12 hours later. The results of the administration of anti-E_2 in this experimental situation are illustrated in Figure 7. Ten IU of PMS induced ovulation in virtually all animals. Treatment with anti-E_2, however, blocked ovulation while treatment with normal sheep serum, or, more importantly, with antibodies to testosterone, had no effect. Treatment with anti-E_2 was not less effective in animals treated with a dose of 45 IU of PMS, a treatment which normally results in superovulation. Results suggest a dose-response relationship between the quantity of anti-E_2 that was administered and the number of animals that ovulated (Fig. 8).

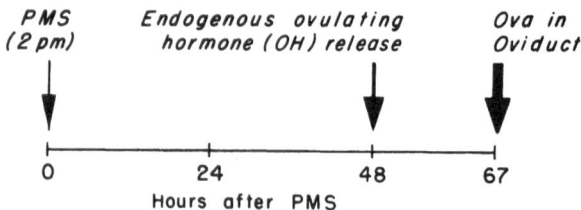

Fig. 6.   Timing of LH release in PMS-treated immature rats.

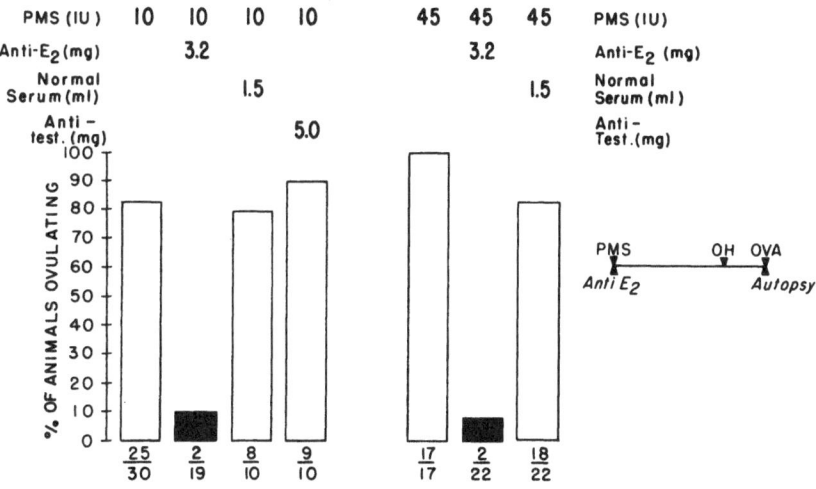

Fig. 7. Effects of anti-E₂ on ovulation in rats treated with 10 or 45 IU of PMS. All rats were injected with 3.2 mg antibody at the same time as with PMS, and were autopsied 67 hours after the PMS injection. Control animals were injected with PMS and either normal sheep serum or antiserum to testosterone.

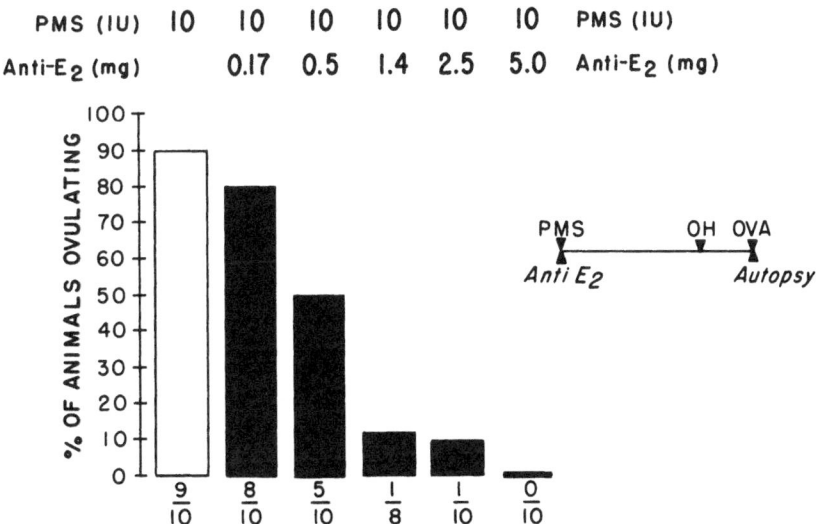

Fig. 8. Effects of increasing amounts of anti-E₂ on ovulation in rats treated with 10 IU of PMS. (Anti-E₂ was injected at the same time as PMS and autopsy was performed 67 hours after the PMS injection.)

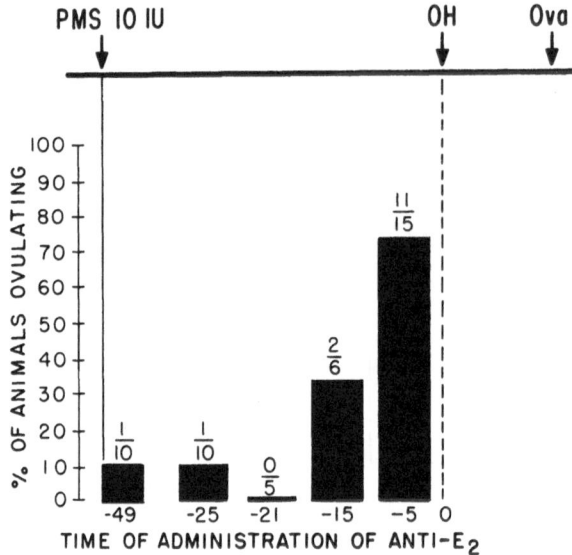

Fig. 9. Effects of time of administration of anti-E₂ on ovulation in rats treated with 10 IU of PMS. (All rats received 3.2 mg of antibody and were autopsied 67 hours after the PMS injection.)

Amounts as small as 0.5 mg of antibody resulted in a 50 percent decrease in the number of ovulations.

It was of interest to determine how long the administration of anti-E_2 could be postponed and still block ovulation (Fig. 9). When the administration of antibody was postponed until 15 hours before the time at which LH discharge would normally occur, there was still almost complete inhibition of ovulation. However, when the antibody was withheld until 5 hours before this critical · period, most of the rats ovulated, indicating that by this time the triggering effect of estrogens upon LH release had already been set in motion.

The Adult Cyclic Rat

The timing of the most important events in the cycle of the 4-day cyclic adult rat is schematically shown in Figure 10. The LH surge occurs

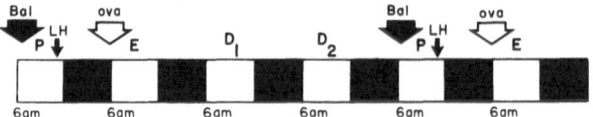

Fig. 10. Timing of ballooning (Bal), LH release (LH), and ovulation (ova) in 4-day cycling rats. P = proestrus; E = estrus; D_1 = first day of diestrus; D_2 = second day of diestrus.

in the afternoon of the day of proestrus, the exact timing of the surge depending upon the day-night schedule in the laboratory. In our laboratory, where the lights are turned on at 6 a.m. for a span of 10 hours, the critical period during which LH can be released lasts from 2 to 5 p.m. The LH discharge is preceded by a rise in the estrogens in the ovarian vein as well as in the peripheral vein blood, as was recently shown by Yoshinaga et al. (1969). This increase in the estrogen levels is accompanied by an increase in uterine weight and a very typical ballooning of the uterus, due to accumulation of fluid in the cavity. Following LH release, progesterone and progesterol levels increase, producing a relaxation of the cervical sphincter (Armstrong, 1968). The fluid is released from the uterus and the ballooning disappears. Ovulation occurs 12 hours after the LH release, 2 days of diestrus follow, and the cycle starts over again.

A study of the effect of the administration of anti-E_2 upon this sequence of events has been reported (Ferin et al., 1969a) and some of the results are illustrated in Figure 11. Twenty-eight control animals were observed during one or more consecutive cycles, and in all, the events followed the pattern illustrated in Figure 10. The experimental group consisted of 28 animals and the antibodies were administered at 10 a.m. of diestrus-2. In 2 of the 28 animals, the administration did not interfere with the normal menstrual cycle, but in the remaining 26, ovulation was postponed by one or more days. In these animals ballooning of the uterus was absent on the morning of proestrus, indicating that the activity of

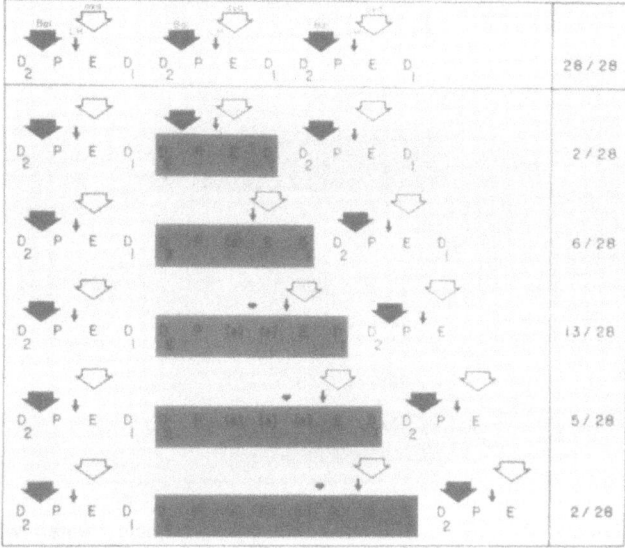

Fig. 11. Effects of anti-E_2 on uterine ballooning and time of ovulation (See Fig. 10 for explanation of abbreviations.)

the circulating estrogens was being suppressed. Deficient estrogen activity was also evident from the vaginal smears which showed only leukocytes on the following morning, at a time when only cornified cells should have been found. In six animals, ovulation was postponed by 24 hours, and in the other animals ovulation was delayed up to 96 hours. The occurrence of ovulation was preceded by signs of renewed estrogen activity such as ballooning of the uterus or the reappearance of cornified cells in the vaginal smear. In all animals the cycle following the experimental cycle was completely normal.

In order to demonstrate that the lack of ovulation was indeed due to the absence of an LH release and that the ovarian response to gonadotropins was not blocked by the treatment with anti-E_2, animals given anti-E_2 were injected with HCG at 2 p.m. on the day of proestrus. This is approximately the time of the endogenous LH release in untreated animals. The administration of 10 IU of HCG produced ovulation in all animals (Fig. 12). In a few cases it has been possible to measure LH levels by radioimmunoassay through the courtesy of Dr. R. Midgley at the University of Michigan. These studies conclusively proved that in animals treated with anti-E_2, ovulation was postponed by a delay in the LH release. Further proof for the role of estrogens in triggering of the pre-

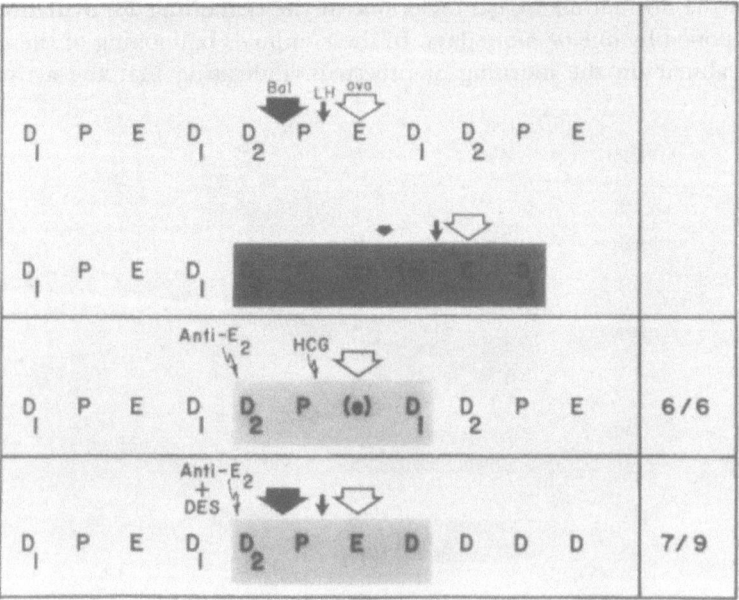

Fig. 12. Effects of HCG or DES on ovulation in animals treated with 5 mg of anti-E_2 at 10 a.m. of diestrus-2. HCG (10 IU) was administered at proestrus (2 p.m.). DES (10 μg) was administered on diestrus-2 (10 a.m.).

ovulatory LH release was obtained in experiments in which DES was administered to animals in which ovulation had been blocked by anti-E$_2$. Since the estrogenic activity of DES is not inhibited by anti-E$_2$, it should be possible to restore ovulation in animals treated with anti-E$_2$ (Fig. 12). A dose of 10 µg of DES administered simultaneously with anti-E$_2$ (but at a different site) restored ovulation in seven out of nine animals.

Since several reports indicate that progesterone may also serve to trigger LH release (Nallar et al., 1966; Zarrow and Hurlbut, 1967), it was of interest to study the effect of anti-P upon ovulation in the cyclic adult rat. Figure 13 illustrates a set of experiments in which anti-P was administered on the morning of diestrus 2, the time at which, in the above described experiments, anti-E$_2$ was given. All animals given anti-P ovulated although the persistence of the uterine ballooning into the morning of proestrus was clear indication that the peripheral effects of progesterone were being suppressed. As mentioned before, the disappearance of the uterine ballooning following the LH surge is a sensitive indicator of the secretion of progesterone.

The results of our studies strongly support the hypothesis that, both in the immature animal treated with PMS, and in the adult cyclic rat, estrogens serve as the trigger that sets off the preovulatory LH release. They do not invalidate the studies in which progesterone has been shown

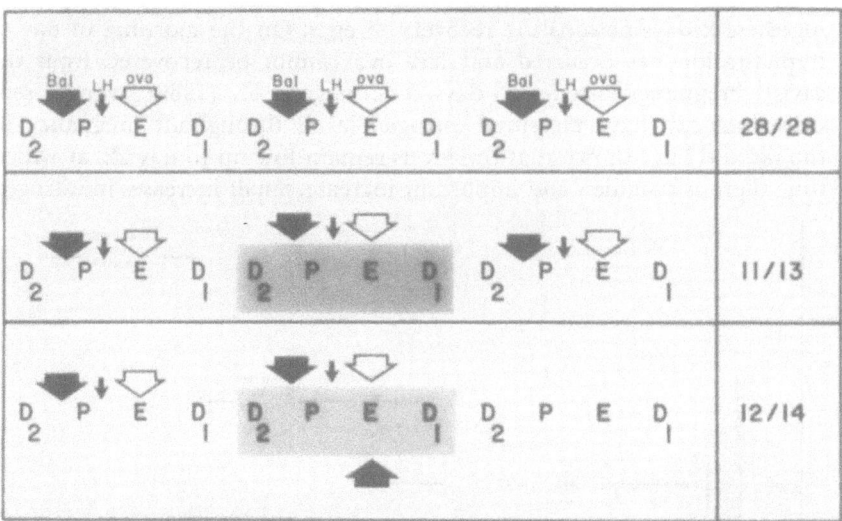

Fig. 13. Effects of normal serum and anti-P on uterine ballooning at proestrus and estrus, and on the time of ovulation. Anti-P was administered on diestrus-2. Upper line = results in untreated controls; Middle line = animals treated with normal serum; Bottom line = animals treated with anti-P. (See Fig. 10 for explanation of abbreviations.)

to produce an LH release, but indicate that this is not the mechanism that operates in the spontaneously cyclic animal. Consistent with this hypothesis are recent studies showing that the level of progesterone increases only after the beginning of the LH surge, and therefore appears to be a consequence rather than a cause of LH release (Kobayashi et al., 1968). Recently, evidence has been presented (Vande Wiele et al., 1970) that in the human also, estrogens initiate the preovulatory LH surge.

STUDIES WITH ANTI-E₂ AND ANTI-P IN THE PREGNANT RAT

Recently we have extended our studies with anti-E_2 and anti-P to the pregnant rat, in an attempt to delineate the role played by estrogens and progresterone during implantation and later stages of pregnancy.

The timing of the events during the early part of pregnancy is schematically represented in Figure 14. Rats are mated in the evening of proestrus. If spermatozoa are present in the vaginal smear on the next day, this day is designated as day 1 of pregnancy. The fertilized ova migrate through the fallopian tubes during days 2 and 3, and enter the uterus on the morning of day 4, remaining free in the uterine cavity until the end of day 5. Flushing of the uterus with physiologic saline during these 2 days permits the recovery of eggs. On the morning of day 6, implantation has occurred and free ova cannot be recovered from the cavity. Pregnancy lasts for 23 days. Yoshinaga et al. (1969), using a sensitive bioassay, have measured estrogen levels throughout pregnancy in the rat and have shown that the levels remain low up to day 22, at which time there is a sudden and important increase. Small increases in estrogen

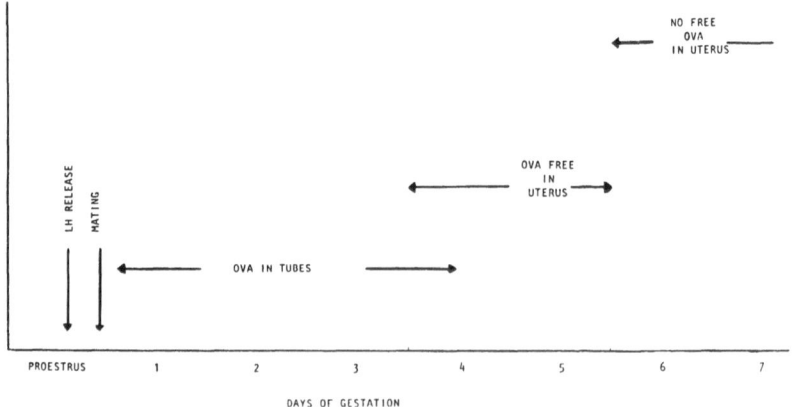

Fig. 14. Timing of nidation in untreated control rats.

concentrations were observed on days 3 and 4, but these levels remained significantly below those observed during proestrus. On the other hand, Hashimoto et al. (1968) have shown that progesterone levels rise early in pregnancy and reach peak values on day 14.

In a series of preliminary experiments, involving only a small number of animals, pregnant rats were injected with anti-E_2 and anti-P on days 3 and 4 to study the effect that inactivation of either progesterone or estrogen activity may have on the time of implantation. The animals were autopsied on days 6 or 7, and the uteri were flushed to check for the presence of free ova (Fig. 15). Free ova were not recovered from the flushings of any of the control animals, autopsied on either day 6 or 7. In

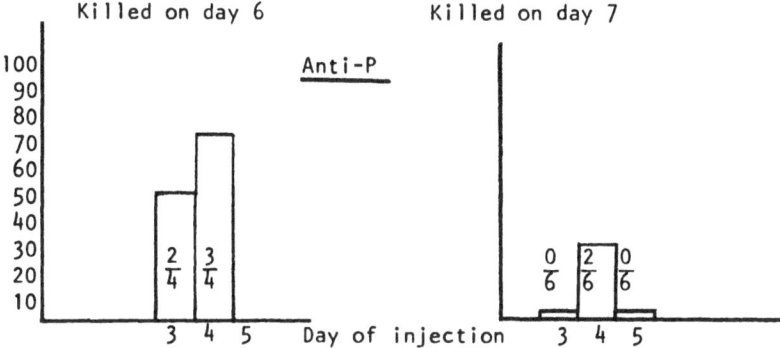

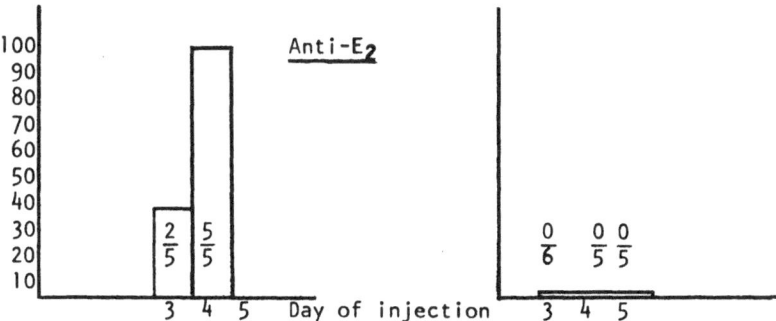

Fig. 15. Percent of treated animals with free intrauterine ova on days 6 and 7 of gestation. A single injection of 10 mg of anti-P or anti-E_2 was given on the day indicated in the bottom of the figure.

contrast, in the animals treated with anti-E_2 or anti-P, free ova could be recovered on these days, indicating that nidation was delayed in both groups.

In a larger group of animals, anti-E_2 and anti-P were administered at various times throughout pregnancy and laparotomies were carried out on days 9, 17 and on the day of delivery. At each time, the number and the size of the implantation sites were recorded. A detailed description of these studies is in preparation (Raziano et al., 1970). The incidence of *complete* resorptions of the conceptus is shown in Figure 16. Most striking and surprising were the results when anti-P was administered on day 11, in which case complete resorption occurred in all animals. These animals started to cycle normally 5 or 6 days after the injection. Anti-P given on days 7 and 15, on the other hand, did not produce complete resorption in any of the treated animals. Two animals were

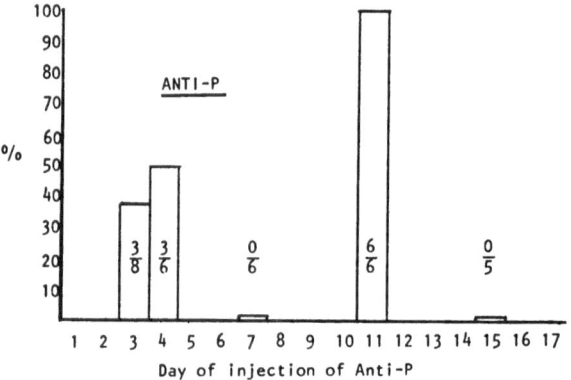

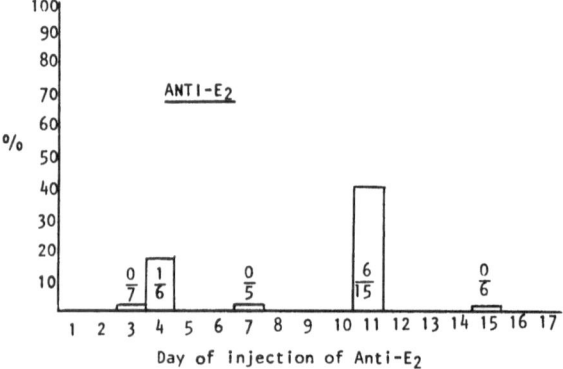

Fig. 16. Percent of animals without implantation sites on day 17 of gestation. A single injection of 10 mg of anti-P or anti-E_2 was given on the day indicated in the bottom of the figure.

injected on day 9 and two animals on day 13, and in each instance the pregnancy continued undisturbed, suggesting that the mid-pregnancy period during which the presence of progesterone is critically important, is of short duration. Anti-E_2 given on day 11 produced complete resorption of the conceptus in 40 percent of the injected animals.

Treatment with anti-E_2 on day 3 resulted in delayed implantation but all the ova that implanted subsequently developed into normal fetuses. On the other hand, administration of anti-P on days 3 and 4 resulted in more profound disturbances, producing complete resorption in half of the treated animals. These results are of special significance since they point to a relationship between disturbances in the hormonal milieu in every pregnancy, and severe complications occurring in the later stages of pregnancy.

REFERENCES

Armstrong, D. T. 1968. Hormonal control of uterine lumen fluid retention in the rat. Amer. J. Physiol., 214:764–771.

Everett, J. W., C. H. Sawyer, and J. E. Markee. 1949. A neurogenic timing factor in control of the ovulatory discharge of luteinizing hormone in the cyclic rat. Endocrinology, 44:234–250.

Ferin, M., P. E. Zimmering, and R. L. Vande Wiele. 1969a. Effects of antibodies to 17β-estradiol on PMS-induced ovulation in immature rats. Endocrinology, 84:893–900.

———— A. Tempone, P. E. Zimmering, and R. L. Vande Wiele. 1969b. Effect of antibodies to 17β-estradiol and progesterone on the estrus cycle of the cat. Endocrinology, 85:1070–1078.

———— P. E. Zimmering, S. Lieberman, and R. L. Vande Wiele. 1968. Inactivation of the biological effects of exogenous and endogenous estrogens by antibodies to 17β-estradiol. Endocrinology, 83:565–571.

Goodfriend, L., and A. H. Sehon. 1961. Antibodies to estrone-protein conjugates II. Endocrinological studies. Canad. J. Biochem. Physiol., 39:961–965.

Hashimoto, I., D. M. Henricks, L. L. Anderson, and R. M. Melampy. 1968. Progesterone and pregn-4-en-20β-ol-3-one in ovarian venous blood during various reproductive states in the rat. Endocrinology, 82:333–341.

Jensen, E. V. 1964. Mechanism of estrogen action in relation to carcinogenesis. *In* Begg, R. W., ed. Canadian Cancer Conference. New York, Pergamon Press, Vol. 6, pp. 145–165.

Kobayashi, F., K. Hara, and T. Miyake. 1968. Luteinizing hormone concentrations in pituitary and in blood plasma during the estrous cycle of the rat. Endocr. Japan., 15:313–319.

Midgley, A. R., Jr., V. Gay, L. Caligaris, R. Rebar, S. Monroe and G. Niswender. 1968. Radioimmunologic studies of rat LH. *In* Rosemberg, E., ed. Gonadotropins, 1968. Los Altos, Geron-X, Inc., pp. 307–312.

Mikhail, G., C. Wu, M. Ferin, and R. L. Vande Wiele. 1970. Radioimmunoassay of plasma estrogens: Use of polymerized antibodies. *In* Péron, F. G., and B. V. Caldwell, eds. Immunologic Methods in Steroid Determination. New York, Appleton-Century-Crofts.

Nallar, R., J. Antunes-Rodrigues, and S. M. McCann. 1966. Effect of progesterone on the level of plasma luteinizing hormone (LH) in normal female rats. Endocrinology, 79:907–911.

Neri, R. O., S. Tolksdorf, S. M. Beiser, B. F. Erlanger, F. J. Agate, Jr., and S. Lieberman. 1964. Further studies on the biological effects of passive immunization with antibodies to steroid-protein conjugates. Endocrinology, 74:593–598.

Raziano, J., A. Tempone, M. Ferin, and R. L. Vande Wiele. 1970. Effects of antibodies to 17β-estradiol and progesterone on nidation and gestation in the rat. (in preparation)

Roy, S., V. B. Mahesh, and R. B. Greenblatt. 1964. Effects of clomiphene on the physiology of reproduction in the rat. III. Inhibition of uptake of radioactive estradiol by the uterus and pituitary gland of immature rat. Acta Endocr., 47:669–675.

Vande Wiele, R. L., J. Bogumil, I. Dyrenfurth, M. Ferin, R. Jewelewicz, M. Warren, T. Rizkallah and G. Mikhail. 1970. Mechanisms regulating the menstrual cycle in women. Recent Progr. Hormone Res., 26: (in press).

Yoshinaga, K., R. A. Hawkins, and J. F. Stocker. 1969. Estrogen secretion by the rat ovary in vivo during the estrous cycle and pregnancy. Endocrinology. 85:103–112.

Zarrow, M. X. and E. L. Hurlbut. 1967. Inhibition and facilitation of PMS-induced ovulation in the immature rat following treatment with progesterone. Endocrinology, 80:735–740.

—— and D. L. Quinn. 1963. Superovulation in the immature rat following treatment with PMS alone and inhibition of PMS-induced ovulation. J. Endocr., 26:181–188.

Zimmering, P. E., S. M. Beiser, and B. F. Erlanger. 1965. Purification and some properties of anti-testosterone antibodies. J. Immunology, 95:262–272.

DISCUSSION

E. KNOBIL. Using the more sensitive methods which we were forced to develop because of the small size and limited blood volume of the rhesus monkey, we have begun to describe the endocrine events within the menstrual cycle in that species. So far we have analyzed nine such cycles. I was interested in Dr. Caldwell's results in the sheep which show a deep decline in plasma LH concentration prior to the surge in response to the administration of estrogen. We have seen this type of decline in LH prior to the surge in just about all of the nine normal cycles we have studied. The ovulatory surge is preceded by several days of a gradual rise in circulating levels of estradiol. The rise becomes very precipitous a day or so before the beginning of the LH surge. Even though the estrogen began to rise before the LH, the estradiol surge is coincident with the LH peak a day before the LH peak. The fall in estradiol is just as precipitous as the fall in preovulatory progesterone, and in the monkey we have established that ovulation occurs at the time of this dip which is a rather reproducible phenomenon in circulating progestins. By laparotomy we have established that this dip is roughly coincident with ovulation. It looks as though progesterone secretion by the preovulatory follicle, as well as estrogen secretion by the preovulatory follicle, is abruptly interrupted just prior to or at the time of ovulation. The estradiol determinations were done on 200 µl of peripheral plasma. The progesterones were done on 500 µl, and the LH determinations on 100 µl. The estradiol and estrone were measured in the method which I referred to briefly in the discussion of Dr. Abraham's paper. The separation technique between free and bound is by dextran coated charcoal. To separate estrone from estradiol we use a simple thin layer chromatographic step on silica gel developing the chromatogram in 95 portions of chloroform to 5 portions of acetone.

N. MOUDGAL. Have any equilibrium dialysis studies been done with regard to the relative ability of estrogens to bind to antibody and uterine-receptor protein? Which has more affinity to bind estradiol?

B. CALDWELL. You want the affinity constant of the receptor protein and the antibody, I believe. The K values for the various antibodies which we have heard described in the past few days differ greatly in magnitude. The Michigan group seems to be fairly certain that its K values are many orders of magnitude greater than the target-tissue protein. The K value of our antibody was determined on the Scatchard plot to be 2.9 x 10^{10} and the binding is extremely tight. If, for example, you add radioactive indicator estradiol to antisera it is virtually impossible to extract it by normal solvent extraction techniques.

N. MOUDGAL. In my laboratory at Bangalore, India, we have been using anti-LH in studies on the role of LH in ovulation and maintenance of pregnancy in the rat. Using PMS-primed rats and HCG or LH as the ovulating hormone, it has been observed that neutralization of HCG or LH during the first two hours after administration results in total inhibition of ovulation. If, however, HCG or LH is allowed to act for a minimum period of 8 hours, administration of the antiserum has no effect. This coincides well with the observation of Dr. Ferin on the effects of anti-estrogen. It may further be pointed out that neutralization of LH during the first 12 days of pregnancy in the rat results in the termination of gestation. Administration of LH antiserum after this day has no effect on the course of pregnancy.

P. Zimmering.   We have done estradiol equilibrium dialysis studies on the receptor protein from ewes. Our measurments were done at 5°C. Receptor proteins, which gave only the 8S peak on sugar gradients, showed quite complex behavior in the equilibrium dialysis system. Two different binding modes were found for estradiol. The binding constants, which represent an average over a wide range of constants that describe cooperative binding, are around 10^6. The data from the second binding mode gave an S-shaped saturation curve. The Scatchard equation does not fit this type of binding. The data were analyzed using the Sips equation, and gave evidence for cooperative or potentiated binding.

W. Leavitt.   Has anyone used the specific radioimmunoassay technique to measure estrogen levels or other steroid levels in tissues, particularly target tissues? With regard to the receptor proteins, I think what has been discussed is the cytosol "receptor." This in fact may be a carrier protein which transports the steroid to effector sites in the target-cell nucleus. Has anyone looked at the nuclear estrogen receptor and the binding affinity of that particular protein? I ask this because the binding affinity of nuclear receptors for estrogen may be similar to that for the estrogen antibody.

W. Odell.   Dr. Korenman, in the Endocrine Division at Harbor General Hospital, has extensively studied the kinetics of binding and affinity of the uterine-binding-receptor protein. The affinity is approximately the same or slightly greater than that of the antisera described at this workshop. Detailed studies of Scatchard plots reveal that the uterine-binding protein (as well as antibodies) does not give a straight-line relationship. At present it appears that there is only one type of binding protein and it is present in both cytoplasm and nucleus and binds estrogens in both locations. Dr. Korenman has developed a highly specific and sensitive competitive-binding assay using this protein and has published several physiologic studies of fluctuations of estradiol in women. The specificity of binding of this protein is different from that described for antibodies to estradiol. It binds *physiologically* active estrogens—stilbestrol is bound more avidly than estradiol. It may thus be used in vitro to study the "estrogenicity" of compounds. Specificity on the binding assay (as for the assays described in this workshop) was achieved by purification of samples on celite columns prior to assay.

S. Gross.   It is best to leave the the C-17 group free in immunoassays as in work with cellular-protein receptors. I would agree with Dr. Zimmering's K_0 value of 10^6. Arithmetic complexity is imparted by performing calculations in a solid-phase system. It is difficult to select end points on a curve.

R. BARNES.   Dr. Ferin, have you had a pathologist look at any of the tissues of your antibody-treated animals?

M. FERIN.   We looked at the ovaries and uteri of immature mice treated with estradiol and anti-estradiol. The changes induced by the estrogen in the ovaries remained unaffected while those in the uterus were nearly completely abolished by the antiserum.

R. BARNES.   This raises a question concerning the tissue of origin. In the target tissue you might not expect to find as much of your antigen or steroid as in the tissue of origin. If you administer antibody it will find the antigen wherever it may be. You have stated that you are selectively affecting steroid without affecting the tissue as you would by ablation of the organ. I would like to put out a word of caution here. Dr. Laurence at the Population Council has studied rats using ovine LH. He found that there were no tissue effects with the antibody to LH in these animals. However, later someone using the same system in rabbits found that there were indeed immunopathologic changes in the pituitary. If we are going to use these antibodies for experimental purposes, particularly with chronic administration, we should take a careful look at the tissues of origin; namely, the pituitary if we are dealing with LH and FSH, and soon, because some things are almost bound to happen. If you look at what might be expected to happen if the antibody attacks the antigen at the tissue of origin, you would have immunopathologic changes there due to a direct attack upon these tissues. I am very much aware of this problem and think we should do localization studies, and also pathologic studies to see what is happening to the tissues of origin.

M. FERIN.   I agree that this problem should be further investigated. However, in the example you cited, one must differentiate between a direct action of the antibody on a tissue and an action due to secondary changes through feedback mechanisms. In the experiments described in this paper, no drastic changes seemed to occur in the ovaries and pituitary, since they were able to respond to repeated administration of HCG and diethylstilbestrol.

K. YOSHINAGA.   I would like to ask about the effect of anti-progesterone on pregnancy. Anti-progesterone was very effective when given on day 11 of pregnancy but not effective on days 9 or 15. If you look at the level of progesterone secretion, it is higher on day 11 of pregnancy than that seen on day 1. How do you explain that you can get the effect of anti-progesterone on day 11 but not on day 9 if anti-progesterone neutralizes progesterone effect? In relation to this question I would like to know if you have done any experiments on the effects of anti-progestin on the gonadotropin secretion, because day 11 is the day when the luteotropic activity of the pituitary is taken over by the placenta.

M. FERIN.   The half-life of these antibodies in rats is of a rather short duration (24 to 48 hours). This would explain why the injection of anti-progesterone on day 9 did not have any effect. This critical period for progesterone on day 11 of pregnancy is indeed of a very short duration, perhaps not longer than 24 hours. We did not measure gonadotropin secretion during the pregnancy. I do not have any explanation for it but can just state the fact that it is of very short duration.

J. W. GOLDZIEHER.   I would like to refer to the slide you had on the effect of testosterone and anti-testosterone on the rat seminal vesicle. I notice that when you gave anti-estrogen as well as testosterone you seemed to get a somewhat greater response than when you gave the testosterone by itself. Was that a significant difference?

M. FERIN.   It was a significant difference.

J. W. GOLDZIEHER.   Perhaps the "physiologic" seminal vesicle response is really the aggregate of both stimulatory (androgenic) and inhibitory (estrogenic) influences. If physiologic, circulating estrogen has an anti-testosterone action you have in this manner removed the estrogenic action and the testosterone shows a full display of its action. This would be a wholly new illustration of the importance of endogenous estrogens in the male.

R. VANDE WIELE.   I would like to come back to this matter of the effect of the antibodies on the tissue. I thought in Dr. Ferin's presentation this question was answered very well. When you give chorionic gonadotropin to these animals they respond normally. If you give them diethylstilbestrol they respond normally. I would say that at least for the length of the experiment that we did, there was definitely no effect of antibodies on the tissue. I think the only effect of the antibodies was by complexing the hapten in the circulation, therefore preventing it from getting into the target organ.

W. ODELL.   As you are aware, in the human castrated or postmenopausal woman, administration of estrogen followed by progestins results in the same kind of LH and FSH discharge that you described, Dr. Caldwell (Odell, W. D., and R. S. Swerdloff, 1968. *Proc. Nat. Acad. Sci., USA,* 61:529). The design of your experiments was pretreatment with progesterone and then a surge of estradiol. In your studies, Dr. Ferin, of course, we do not know in detail the endogenous secretion of the ovaries in terms of progestogen versus estradiol. You have shown that anti-progesterone did not abolish the LH surge. I wonder if you would like to speculate on whether the progestogen has any role in stimulating this surge. Secondly, specifically to you, Dr. Caldwell, have you sequentially administered estrogens alone, without a progestogen, to your castrated animals and given the same surge of LH on top of estrogen? If so, does this produce the same type of LH peak? In other words, is there any requirement for baseline secretion or for fluctuating secretion of progestogens? Both of you mentioned the increases in 17-hydroxyprogesterone which occurs before the ovulatory peak in women.

B. CALDWELL.   In the sheep experiment that we reported, there seemed to be a need for pretreatment with progesterone. However, whether or not the progesterone has any role at all in the release of LH, we do not know, although we are very much involved in experiments designed to provide some answers on this matter.

M. FERIN.   In rats, anti-progesterone, in amounts that inhibited most of the circulating progesterone, did not affect the number of ova released at ovulation. Therefore, one could suppose that the LH surge was identical to that in the normal animal. This evidence does not rule out the possibility of a synergistic effect of very small amounts of progesterone on LH release, but implies that estrogen is the most important if not the only trigger.

W. ODELL.   When one administers estrogen alone to a eugonadal woman, one observes a discharge of LH (Swerdloff, R. S., and W. D. Odell, 1969. *J. Clin. Endocr.*, 29:157) but no increase in FSH. FSH is released concomitantly with the ovulatory peak in women and nobody knows whether it is required at that moment or not.

G. NISWENDER.   I think there is recent evidence in a paper published by Goding et al. (1969) which is pertinent. They have shown that, in an anestrous sheep in which steroids are extremely low, at any time by almost any route of administration of estradiol they were able to induce a substantial and very repeatable LH peak without an apparent need for progesterone involvement.

M. FERIN.   We have done some experiments in PMS-treated rats in which we tried to overcome the blockage of ovulation induced by anti-E_2 by the administration of progesterone. These attempts were successful in that most animals ovulated. However, the number of ova released remained always low (2 to 4).

C. MIGEON.   When one prepares antibodies, let us say for example, estrogen antibodies, does it mean that the immunized animal has for all purposes no biologically active estrogens, since its endogenous hormone is bound to estrogen antibodies? It may not be of great significance that the immunized animal has no biologically active estrogens, but I am wondering about a personal problem with our animals immunized against aldosterone. If steroid antibodies bind and therefore inactivate steroids, then our rabbits might still be able to produce aldosterone, but they would not be able to respond to it. Since in vitro our aldosterone antibodies cross-react with corticosterone, I wonder whether we will end up with Addisonian rabbits.

M. FERIN.   There is an abstract (R. Dusquenoy 1967. 51st Federation Proc. Meeting 26:297) about the effects of active immunization with an estrone-protein conjugate on DMBA-induced mammary carcinoma in rats. The author was hoping to reduce the incidence of tumors but obtained the opposite effect, presumably due to an increase in the production of estrogens via a feedback mechanism.

K. CATT.   May I return to the work mentioned by Dr. Niswender? In those experiments on the anestrous sheep, we gave intramuscular doses of estradiol of 2, 10, and 50 µg. In the animals given 10 µg and more, there followed reproducible LH peaks of large magnitude similar to estrous LH peaks (Goding, J. R., et al. 1969. *Endocrinology*, 85:133) occurring in all animals 8 to 12 hours after the administration of estrogen. When estradiol was given by infusion at a rate of 3 µg per hour, all animals treated in this fashion showed LH peaks after about the same time. More recently, these experiments have been followed by estrogen administration to ovariectomized ewes. These results have shown an initial fall in plasma LH level followed by a large estrus-type peak of LH release.

L. GOODFRIEND.   Did you look at the levels of circulating steroids after administration of the antisera?

M. FERIN.   No. What we know, however, is that basal and cornified cells appear in the vaginal smears 2 days after administration of progesterone in the earlier part of pregnancy. Whether this is due to an increase in secretion of estrogen rather than to the removal of the inhibitory influence of progesterone, we do not know.

L. GOODFRIEND.   These studies in immunoendocrinology have cleared up a 10-year worry, at least for me, because in our early studies on intraperitoneal injection of mixtures of estrogen and anti-estrogen we observed inhibition of the 6-hour uterotrophic effect in immature rats. On the other hand, the Columbia group could not find this early effect either in their initial studies (Lieberman et al., 1959. *Recent Progr. Hormone Res.*, 15:165–196) or in the later studies by Neri et al. (1964. *Endocrinology*, 74:593–598), and there was a bit of mystery about what the antiserum was doing. I believe your studies provide a clear demonstration that what is involved here is the *level* of *circulating* anti-steroid antibodies. If you administer the antibodies by a route that is unfavorable for the rapid development of a high level of circulating anti-steroid antibodies, competition is set up between the steroid you are injecting at some other site for the antibodies which are slowly getting into the circulation, on the one hand, and target sites of the steroid, on the other—and the latter can be favored. If you have high levels of anti-steroid antibodies in the circulation, you prevent the steroid from getting to the target tissue. This leaves open the question of whether or not the steroid-antibody complex is hormonally active, but simply cannot get to the target site. Perhaps in vitro systems incorporating steroid and anti-steroid antibody could throw light on this question.

M. FERIN.   In the experiments shown in Chapter 11, Figure 1, in which the uterotrophic effect of estradiol is inhibited by anti-E_2, we can see that the uterine weight never completely reverted to that of the controls. This, we thought, was due to the action of some unbound estrogen. But this could also be due to hormonal activity of the steroid-antibody complex. We do not know the answer and experiments should be carried out to clarify this point.

M. HARPER.   In those rats to which you gave the antiserum to estradiol and prevented implantation, was this a total inhibition or did you in fact study these animals further to see if implantation occurred subsequently? In other words just as you delayed ovulation in your cycling rats, did the same thing apply to the implantation process?

M. FERIN.   Implantation, just as LH release, was indeed delayed by about 24 hours when anti-E_2 was given prior to nidation. However, most of the ova implanted. When given later in the pregnancy, anti-E_2 was much less effective than anti-P in interrupting the pregnancy, pointing out the relative smaller role of estrogens.

M. HARPER.   In connection with determining exactly what you are doing with these antisera to steroids, I presume that you have not in fact looked at what the antiserum to estradiol might do to implantation in the hamster or the rabbit. We know that in these species if you remove the ovaries shortly after ovulation and give progesterone alone, implantation occurs quite normally. It might be interesting from this point of view to see, if you give antiserum to estradiol to hamsters before implantation (on day 3, for instance), whether implantation takes place at the normal time.

B. CALDWELL.   We did just that, Dr. Harper, and we found no effect whatsoever on pregnancy in 12 hamsters studied, using both active and passive immunization procedures. This confirms that estradiol in the hamster is probably not essential to the maintenance of pregnancy.

A. MUNCK.   Now that the cause-and-effect relationships between the estrogen peak and later events is becoming clearer, I wonder if you have ideas on the question of the estrogen peak itself—what causes its rise and its rapid decay?

W. ODELL.   There is now some suggestive evidence from the treatment of hypophysectomized humans and infertile humans that, once you initiate the sequence of events leading to follicular development and growth by FSH, these events may then take place independent of pituitary secretion. During follicle development, rising estrogen levels may be a resultant of the developing follicle which in turn is perhaps at least partially independent of FSH secretion once initiated. This rising estrogen secretion may then trigger the LH peak when follicle maturation has occurred. The event that follows that LH surge, in the ovary, is ovulation. Perhaps that event is itself somehow associated with the observed fall in estrogen secretion, and corpus luteum function is then associated with the secondary rise.

R. VANDE WIELE.   In Recent Progress in Hormone Research, Volume 26, I have presented a hypothesis to explain the rise in estrogens in the preovulatory phase in the female. The striking observation is that when FSH is either decreasing, or at best constant, there occurs the maximum rate of increase in estrogen secretion. If hypophysectomized women are given constant doses of FSH in plasma you get the same curve seen in the normal preovulatory phase. The hypothesis I presented was that once the follicle starts to grow, it starts making estrogens and androgens and the ultimate control of the follicle and secretion is not so much via the level of FSH but due to a positive effect of the estrogens on the growth of the follicle and the effect of the androgens. This is based on animal work for which confirmation in humans will be necessary.

C. LONGCOPE.   In collaboration with the Worcester group, I measured the concentration of radioactivity as estradiol and estrone in whole blood following the injection of ^{3}H-estradiol-17β into an immunized sheep. The disappearance of ^{3}H-estradiol-17β was very slow with a single half-life of about 280 minutes. In comparison, the disappearance of ^{3}H-estradiol-17β in the normal sheep can be expressed as the sum of two experiments with indices of 4 and 40 minutes respectively. The antibody, which may be reasonably specific under controlled conditions in the test tube, is not quite so specific in the animal, where concentrations of steroid and antibody are far different, since the estrone formed from estradiol and measured in the blood as estrone also was strongly bound and disappeared very slowly.

E. ROSEMBERG.   I wish to come back to the question relating to the influence of estrogens produced by a stimulated follicle upon release of pituitary LH. Drs. Odell and Vande Wiele referred to the temporal events occurring during the administration of exogenous gonadotropins which were specifically referred to as FSH. It is important to remember that, during the proliferative phase of the menstrual cycle, the circulating plasma levels of FSH and LH as measured by radioimmunoassays in normal women show a relationship in that these two hormones are present at a certain ratio. Studies related to the excretion of FSH and LH during the menstrual cycle have revealed similar findings. Hence, during the proliferative phase of the menstrual cycle, the ovarian follicle is probably stimulated by both FSH and LH. It is important to realize that the only available preparations of human gonadotropins used so far have been those prepared from the urine of postmenopausal women, which contain both FSH and LH. Precise information concerning the effect of FSH upon the ovary will be gained only when purified human pituitary FSH will be available for investigation. Until then, I doubt that we can make statements regarding the effect of the so-called "FSH" administered in the form of mixtures of gonadotropins upon follicular development and steroidogenesis. What makes the follicle produce estrogen and turn on all of these mechanisms? Dr. Ferin and Dr. Vande Wiele referred to the effect of administration of exogenous gonadotropins you referred to as administration of FSH. I think we all have to realize that in the proliferative phase of the cycle, studying normal women, there is a certain measurable relationship in plasma as well as urine, a relationship of FSH and LH, a certain ratio of these two hormones. I think more precise information will be gained when we administer purified human pituitary FSH. Until then I doubt if we can make real statements and comparisons with parenterally administered gonadotropins that are really mixtures.

W. ODELL.   Another word of caution on the antisera studies. From the polypeptide immunoassay areas there is evidence that specificity studies in radioimmunoassays and studies of biologic neutralization give very different ideas of antiserum specificity. For example, a series of purified hormones may fail to cross-react in a specific radioimmunoassay. Then if one looks at the antisera in a totally different way, either their ability to neutralize the biologic activities of the hormones that failed to react in the immunoassay or the ability of the antisera to bind the hormone in the labeled form, may find by both means that the antisera indeed do cross-react. Failure in the steroid immunoassays to show cross-reactions with various steroids, therefore, is not full evidence that these antisera when used for neutralizing might not neutralize some other steroidal substances. Neutralization studies of the kind Dr. Ferin reported, wherein biologic activity is neutralized, are important documents. Further studies should show evidence that the biologic activities of other steroids are also not affected.

SUMMARY

William D. Odell

Division of Endocrinology
Harbor General Hospital
Torrance, California

In these three days under an intimate stimulating environment with free interchange of information, we have concerned ourselves with immunologic means of quantifying steroid hormones. Ten years ago Berson and Yalow (1959) and Ekins (1960) first published the principles of competitive binding assays. Since that time the general applicability of these principles has become evident; the procedures may be adopted to quantify any hormonal substance. Experience gained by many investigators in characterizing competitive binding assays for polypeptides has led to increased comprehension of the required properties of such systems (Odell et al., 1969). Antisera have been prepared against progressively smaller hormones: ACTH (MW 4566), gastrin (MW 2096), vasopressin (MW 1080), and angiotensin II (MW 1170). Even though so-called antigenic determinants are believed to be approximately equivalent to 600 to 800 molecular weight substances, smaller haptenic substances have been shown to be capable of being immunogenic, usually when coupled to larger molecules. Thus in the past few years, antibodies have been prepared against steroid-protein conjugates and the steroids themselves have served as haptenic reactants (Erlanger et al., 1957). Several important properties of antisera are of concern to us.

Specificity

Antisera prepared against polypeptide hormones show great variation in specificity from animal to animal, and from time to time within the same animal. Experience has shown that specificity must be exhaustively and precisely defined. We have seen here at this workshop that similar

problems exist with antisera directed against steroids. Although Drs.
Niswender and Midgley showed specificity could be in part directed
by appropriate selection of the site of conjugation of steroid to protein,
the studies of the other groups demonstrated variation in specificity.
Specificity of antisera used in steroid immunoassays thus must also be
rigorously tested.

Titer

The titer of antisera used for polypeptide hormones over 20,000 in
molecular weight is usually in the range of 1:100,000 to 1:10,000,000 dilution. The most frequently immunized animals have been guinea pigs,
rabbits, and chickens. For polypeptides under 5,000 molecular weight,
antisera are in general more difficult to prepare; conjugation frequently,
but not invariably, has been required. Titers have tended to be lower.
For the steroid antisera discussed here, it appears both rabbits and sheep,
but not guinea pigs, have produced satisfactory results. There is not sufficient comparative data from a single investigative group for one to conclude either species is superior. Niswender and Midgley had eminent success immunizing rabbits; the other groups appeared to favor sheep.
Titers generally have been lower than those observed after immunization
with larger polypeptides.

Affinity

The association constant of antisera may be described by the
equation:

$$K = \frac{K_1}{K_2} = \frac{[H \cdot Ab]}{[H] [Ab]}$$

where $H \cdot Ab$ = hormone-antibody complex, $[H]$ = free hormone, and
$[Ab]$ = free antibody.

When data from polypeptide antigen-antibody reactions are plotted
on a Scatchard plot, a linear relationship is not observed, and a series
(not one) of association constants may be calculated (Odell et al., 1969).
Using this or similar techniques, affinity constants have been presented
during this symposium for steroid-antibody interactions, for the most
part from data collected with solid-phase binding of the antisera. It was
pointed out in discussion that all the reactants in the association reaction
are expressed as molar concentrations of these substances *in solution*. But
an antiserum bound to solid phase is not in solution. Thus this equation
may not be adequate to describe solid-phase systems, and association constants may not be directly comparable to those estimated for the same

antiserum with reactants in solution. In theory, the concentration of the antibodies is very high just at the surface of the solid phase, but one millimeter away it is zero. In general, affinity of antisera may be correlated with the sensitivity possible with an assay system.

Dr. Abraham demonstrated that the binding affinities of 6,7 ^{3}H-estradiol and 2,4,6,7 ^{3}H-estradiol for one antiserum were different; apparently the alterations in ring A produced by substituted tritium was sufficient to decrease antibody binding. The complexity of antigen-antibody interactions and variations with different antisera is demonstrated, however, by comparing these observations of ^{3}H-estradiol with data presented by Drs. Niswender and Midgley; radioiodinated methyl-ester-tyrosine-steroid conjugates and radioiodinated bovine serum albumin-steroid conjugates appeared to react *equally* or *superior* to non-conjugated tritiated steroids. The alterations in steroid size and configuration are much greater with these conjugates than with tritium labeling.

Methods of Separating Antibody Bound from Free Hormone

For polypeptide hormone radioimmunoassays a great variety of separation techniques have been used. General categories have included physical, chemical, and immunologic means. Techniques described here for steroid immunoassays have included solid-phase techniques, double-antibody techniques, charcoal, and dextran-gel. Solid-phase techniques described at this symposium have all been, thus far, adsorption of the antibodies to plastic, a process affected by pH, molarity, and temperature. shown, protein concentration of the incubating solutions exposed to As Dr. Catt (Catt et al., 1968 and Catt, 1969) and many others have coated solid-phase materials influences the amount of antibody bound, and antibody adsorption is usually not completely irreversible in incubating solutions of widely differing protein concentrations. Thus, if protein solutions such as unextracted serum are to be assayed using solid-phase separation techniques, the protein content of all tubes must be carefully controlled. Actual chemical bonding of antisera to solid-phase media as described by Wide and Porath (1966) may offer advantages.

Assay Procedures

None of the antisera described appear to be capable of quantifying a single steroid in unextracted serum or plasma with complete reliability. Hopefully, this may one day be possible, thus greatly simplifying measurement. At present, all steroid immunoassay systems described here at this workshop require the extraction and separation or purification of the steroid prior to assay. Several speakers have emphasized the importance of proper purification and cleansing of reagents used for separation techniques; significant interference with the antigen-antibody detection systems and problems of high blanks were described. Another important reason for extracting steroid hormones prior to measurement must be emphasized. Competitive binding reactions take place with every binding protein present. Resultant assay curves represent complex interrelations of (1) a variety of antibodies, (2) steroid binding of α- or β-globulins, and (3) albumin in both the samples to be assayed and the antisera if used in large concentrations. It is probably wisest to remove all such *non-antibody, steroid-binding proteins* prior to assay by extraction and purification.

In spite of these many points of concern, steroid radioimmunoassays are practical, sufficiently sensitive, and with care, sufficiently specific to permit quantitation in serum of humans and animals. Abraham showed good agreement with steroid measurements by other techniques. The great advantages over the laborious double-isotope-derivative assay procedures, developed and perfected and painfully used by many illustrious members of this audience, are readily apparent. The immunoassays are very much simpler and may be applied to smaller samples.

The use of the assay systems and the exploitation of specific binding properties for neutralization studies to gain insights into additional physiologic roles of each steroid hormone has been described this morning by Dr. Caldwell and co-workers and Dr. Ferin and co-workers. Clarification of the possible role of preovulatory increases in estradiol in inducing the LH surge was offered. There is no doubt that the techniques described, amplified, and clarified during these days will find progressively widespread use. Hopefully the frank and extended interchange at this workshop will hasten the spread of these techniques to investigators throughout the world.

REFERENCES

Berson, S. A., and R. S. Yalow. 1959. Assay of plasma insulin in human subjects by immunological methods. Nature (London), 184:1648.

Catt, K. J. 1969. Discussion following radioimmunoassay with antibody-coated discs and tubes. Karolinska Symposia on Research Methods in Reproductive Endocrinology, 1st Symposium, Immunoassay of Gonadotrophins.

———— H. D. Niall, G. W. Tregear, and H. G. Burger, 1968. Disc solid-phase radioimmunoassay of human luteinizing hormone. J. Clin. Endocr., 28:121.

Ekins, R. P. 1960. The estimation of thyroxine in human plasma by an electrophoretic technique. Clin. Chim. Acta, 5:453–459.

Erlanger, B. F., F. Borek, S. M. Beiser, and S. Lieberman. 1957. Steroid-protein conjugates. I. Preparation and characterization of conjugates of bovine serum albumin with testosterone and with cortisone. J. Biol. Chem., 228:713.

Odell, W. D., G. Abraham, H. Raud, R. S. Swerdloff, and A. Fisher. 1969. Influence of immunization procedures on the titer, affinity, and specificity of antisera to glycopolypeptides. Acta Endocrinol, Suppl., 142:54.

Wide, L., and J. Porath. 1966. Radioimmunoassay of proteins with the use of Sephadex-coupled antibodies. Biochim. Biophys. Acta, 130:257.

INDEX